Praise for
*More of You: The Fat Girl's Field
Guide to the Modern World*

"Existing in a world that constantly tells you what you should be, what you should do, and how you should look is hard, frustrating, and terrifying, especially if you exist in a non-normative, *fat* body. Beck's *More of You* gives readers the language and tools to reframe our bodies not merely as objects designed to get us from point A to point B, but as sacred creations, designed for existing in relationship and with love and passion for justice for *all* bodies. Following this field guide helps readers to understand fat within the context of oppression, accessibility, and disability and reframe the discussion in important ways."

—Dianna E. Anderson, author of
Damaged Goods, *Problematic*, and *In Transit*

"In *More of You: The Fat Girl's Field Guide to the Modern World*, Amanda Martinez Beck sets out to give the reader a knapsack of tools to navigate a world that is often an unsafe and unjust place for fat people. With her characteristic wit and empathy, Martinez Beck gives an excellent overview of the history of fat activism, as well as vital key points, or touchstones, that she has gleaned about her body and her life, including her signature line, 'All bodies are good bodies.' This book is a must-read for anyone with a body."

—Jessica Kantrowitz, author of
The Long Night, *365 Days of Peace*, and
Blessings for the Long Night

"Beck's religion informs her writing as she reconciles being a person of size with being one of faith, taking up space in a society that wants fat women to shrink and mingling the body's inherent goodness with pain and discrimination. This book is a fat liberation manifesto that recognizes the gains of the past—and the fights of tomorrow."

—Lindley Ashline, body acceptance photographer and activist

"Intricately weaving personal storytelling and pieces of the Christian Scriptures, this book meets us at the intersection of the fat liberation movement and our faith, opening our minds and hearts to this truth: God's love isn't contingent on your weight, body size, or body shape."

—Patrilie Hernandez, body liberation advocate and founder of Embody Lib

"Practical and straightforward with beautiful prose and a message of hope and freedom. Beck offers helpful tools for navigating a world designed to exclude fat people. She weaves together the strands of self-advocacy, history of the fat liberation movement, intersectional justice, and compelling memoir to provide a guidebook for all of us who want to live in such a way that we are at home in our body and in this world."

—J. Nicole Morgan, author of
*Fat and Faithful: Learning to Love
Our Bodies, Our Neighbors, and Ourselves*

"Beck walks us through ways to relate to, care for, and appreciate our bodies as they are this very day. She includes information about the history of fat activism that will inspire and give hope to everyone."

—Lisa Du Breuil, LICSW, fat activist,
and clinical social worker

MORE

OF

YOU

MORE OF YOU

THE FAT GIRL'S FIELD GUIDE TO THE MODERN WORLD

AMANDA MARTINEZ BECK

Broadleaf Books

MINNEAPOLIS

MORE OF YOU
The Fat Girl's Field Guide to the Modern World

The author is represented by WordServe Literary Group, www.wordserveliterary.com.

Cover design: FaceOut Studios

Print ISBN: 978-1-5064-7424-3
eBook ISBN: 978-1-5064-7425-0

Printed in Canada

DEDICATION

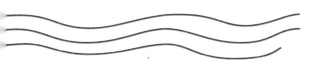

This book is dedicated to J. Nicole Morgan, whose work impacted every part of it. Thank you for leading by saying, "I'll go first."

CONTENTS

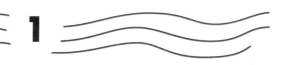

1

ALL BODIES ARE GOOD BODIES

Good: to be desired or approved of; the quality of something that fulfills its purpose.

I LIVE MY LIFE IN A LARGER BODY. I have swallowed the shame of not finding anything to wear when my friends have new and formfitting clothes. I have experienced the embarrassment of literally not fitting in, both in the child-sized amusement park rides and the seats of friends' cars. And I have been subjected to countless doctors' assumptions and prejudices about me and my body, including that I am lazy or lying about what I have eaten. For literal decades, all I wanted to do was shrink so that I could fully participate in the life around me that I saw all my not-fat friends enjoy, seemingly so easily. All I wanted was to conform to the impossible demands of the culture around me that says in order to be worthy—to be good—I had to make myself smaller. It never occurred to me that maybe it wasn't my body that needed to change but the culture itself.

After over twenty years of trying to change my body and make it smaller and more culturally compliant, the wave of discontentment swelling in my soul reached tidal proportions.

I knew that if I gave myself permission, that wave could come down on all I thought I had known about bodies—about how they were "supposed" to look and function. If I let it, that wave would come and clear the path ahead of me, setting me free to live my life in the body I inhabited right at that moment. I decided to let it crash and tear down all the scaffolding of shame and other people's expectations. I didn't know what my life would look like afterward, but I was tired of trying so hard to placate the siren of "thinness and health" that called so loudly.

As this wave crashed down on the assumptions and expectations I had internalized about bodies, I came across a phrase that latched onto my heart and would not let go: *all bodies are good bodies*. At first, I balked. The statement was so simple and yet so broad. I wanted it to be true because, deep down inside, I yearned for goodness, not just for my body but for all of me. If all bodies were good, that meant my body—large, weak, and imperfect—was good too. I didn't know if I could ever believe that, but I wanted to.

"What makes a thing good?" This question swirled in my head for a while, and I turned to the wisdom of the ancients to make sense of it. Aristotle taught that a thing is good that fulfills its purpose. So if I wanted to determine whether *any* body was good, I first needed to understand what the purpose of a body was. Before the wave of discontent had enlightened my framework for understanding bodies, I had assumed that the purpose of my body was to be perfect. That perfection was made up of thinness and health, free from the weaknesses of fatness and illness. But as a Christian, and specifically as a Catholic, when I started to drill down into this concept of perfection, I found that it contradicted what I knew to be true about the God who has a human body, Jesus.

First, I was pretty sure that God created humans with bodies to have a relationship with his people, not to show them off as perfect specimens. Moreover, I had learned that flawlessness wasn't the aim of the Christian life; rather, the aim is a relationship with God through Jesus. All the cultural rules I knew about what bodies *should* be like started to remind me of the fastidious record-keeping for which Jesus blasted some religious leaders. Perhaps most importantly, after the crucifixion and resurrection of Jesus, his resurrected body isn't what we would call perfect. In fact, Jesus uses the scars of his love to identify himself. In Revelation, we read that Jesus is the Lamb standing as if he has been slain. The resurrected God-man walks with a limp.

Seeing all this, I came to the conclusion that the purpose of my body wasn't perfection or thinness but a relationship with God and with my neighbor as myself. Any body—no matter its size, ability, or level of health—can have a deep and meaningful relationship with God and with others. All this being true, I knew I could confidently say that yes, all bodies are good bodies.

All bodies are good bodies because the purpose of a body is relationship, not perfection. In the years since I discovered these truths, my world has been turned upside down—and let me tell you, my world needed a good shake-up. Shame about my body size, guilt over my inability to make myself smaller, and fear of the future started to peel away, revealing the little girl inside of me who just needed someone to speak tenderly to her. As I began to speak tenderly to her—to my inner self—healing started to flow. Now that little girl knows she doesn't have to hide herself, and together we can be the fully integrated person I was created to be.

On the journey toward healing and wholeness, another truth solidified in my mind: *My body is good today.* Wow. Really? My body, just as it is *today*, is good? This one was harder to swallow. I could believe on a theoretical level that all bodies were good, but like everyone around me, I had been swimming in the waters of body discontentment for so long that I didn't know how to *be* if I weren't striving to change my body and make it better. To think that my current body was good undermined so much of my daily reality. If my body is good right now, I don't have to stress about changing it. If my fat body is good right now, it means I'm worth as much as the thin lady next to me and as the man in a wheelchair in front of us. I can just *be* in my body. I don't have anything to prove. I don't have to perform. I don't have to be different than I am.

My *today body* is good because the purpose of my body is relationship—not perfection. This truth is a revolution in my soul, upending the dictatorship of diet culture and restoring *the way things were always meant to be.* In a world filled with injustice and unthinkable pain, believing in a good God, a God who loves each of us and has a purpose for our lives, is a legitimate challenge. In one sense, it's easy for me to believe. I grew up in a well-off, well-educated white family in a place of nearly unparalleled privilege. And yet I had so often been told—in spoken and unspoken ways—that my body wasn't good enough. This book is my attempt at peeling back my experience with fatness, dissecting it, and analyzing it so that I can give guidance to others who have experiences similar to mine. This is not a definitive guide for what it means to be fat, because that experience is so beautiful, painful, and varied—in America alone, to say nothing of the wider world—that no book could contain it. And in the process of finding my own voice, I have learned that there are layers of oppression and that when they overlap, oppression is compounded.[1] The struggles of others less privileged and more oppressed than me are stories I treasure because they are the lived experiences of dear people in good bodies. So to my Black readers, my LGBTQ readers, my transgender readers, my disabled readers— thank you for your patience as I unpack my pain and share what I've learned as a fat, white, cisgender, straight woman. I know I don't speak for everyone, and I am thankful for your correction along the way.

HOW TO USE THIS BOOK

Each chapter in this book includes a few things: an entry for the fat lexicon (available in its entirety in appendix A), items to add to the packing list for our journey (full list in appendix B), and a touchstone to put in your pocket along the way (the titles of every chapter). Some words in the lexicon may be new terms to you, while others are familiar words with new definitions. Items on the packing list are for your quick reference after you've read the chapter and then the book in its entirety; they are practical tools to help while you're living your best fat life out in the field.

The touchstones are like mantras to meditate on and remind yourself of daily, letting the truth they contain take root deep in your soul. I think of each of these as a message etched on a small rock that I carry with me. When I feel it inside my pocket, I recall the words imprinted on it and grow stronger on the way.

Thanks for reading. I'm excited and honored to be on this journey with you. Ready to get going?

PACKING LIST

- Knapsack
- Sturdy hiking shoes
- Clothing with pockets
- Open heart and mind

TOUCHSTONE

ALL BODIES ARE GOOD BODIES.

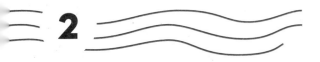

And indeed, it was very good.
Genesis 1:31

2

YOUR TODAY BODY IS GOOD

Body positivity: originally used by fat liberationists as shorthand for their work, today it has been co-opted by non-fat people and corporations as a focus on feeling good about your body rather than focusing on freeing people from anti-fat oppression.

I'VE BEEN A FAT ACTIVIST FOR MANY YEARS, but I still get nervous about other people's perceptions of my body. When I walk into a room, I'm always bringing more of me, in a culture that demands that I make myself smaller and bring less of me to the table. I walk into a room, and I come to a table that doesn't look like it was built for someone my size. I come with a big body, a personality that won't let me sit idly by when I see injustice around me, and a purple cane or ruby-red wheeled walker to help me get from place to place (depending on the day and the severity of my pain). And in every room I enter, I find chairs that won't hold me. What am I supposed to do? My subconscious immediately plays the What Will They Think of my Body? game (zero out of five stars—do *not* recommend), and I find myself engaging the very scary proposition that I—both my body and my being—am too much for the people around me.

It's hard in a culture that continually pushes us toward its concept of self-improvement, urging us to transform our *today bodies*—exactly as our bodies are today—into some wildly healthy and thin future bodies. That costs time, money, and energy that most of us don't have. So we look at our today bodies in the mirror and feel helpless and hopeless, wondering how we will ever be able to make our bodies good enough. It's like we're on a journey, and, unsure of the way, we stumble, fall, and hurt ourselves.

Genesis begins with a creation story that describes God as good, the world that God created as good, and the humans God created as very good. But what does that really mean for us? For starters, it means that our bodies are good. And if you object to that concept because of what comes next in the story—or what you've been told about what comes next in the story, which is often called "the Fall" in Christian theology—when Adam and Eve's disobedience in the garden of Eden ushered in pain, sickness, acrimony, disease, and death, then I challenge you to get outside and soak up some Mother Nature. I live in Texas, where it is hotter than proverbial hell in the summer, but even I can sit on my back stoop in the cool of the morning and watch the earth bustle with its goodness all around me. The pair of alpha robins battling for prominence. The squirrels nibbling the seeds and nuts they've found in the freshly mown grass. New life taking root literally anywhere—like the little green sprout that has taken up residence in my gutter's silt. This earth is good, and its goodness feeds my soul.

All this goodness—of our earth and our God and our bodies—fuels the imagination. Every time we bump into something, whether through text or screen or canvas or relationship, it scatters its seed onto the garden of our soul. These things can take root and grow into salvation, flowering into justice. Somewhere along the way (let's be honest, it was probably thanks to C. S. Lewis because I'm basic), a seed of glory rooted itself in the deepest part of me. In his book *The Great Divorce*, Lewis's narrator boards a bus, invited to leave the hellish gray city for the foothills of heaven. Along the way, the narrator encounters several travelers who will not leave behind their childish obsessions and competitions. Their resistance to going further up and further in is farcical—their foolishness is seen by everyone but themselves. Because they fail to let go of the shadows that must fall away in order to travel into glory, true life—a glorious life full of light and joy—evades them. The bus pulls up to the station at the base of the heavenly mountains, and the riders disembark. The narrator marvels at a person apparently approaching them: a woman whose very essence of life pours out of her, spilling over and onto the animal entourage who delight in her presence. The hell of the gray town and the greed, fear, and insecurity of the travelers were a shadow of reality. But that woman, she was *real*. "You desire truth in my inmost being," from Psalm 51, became a fervent prayer as I began to imagine how I could be like her, soaked in goodness.

The image of this woman as described by Lewis imprinted in my mind, and I knew—in that deep but a-rational knowing way—that such beauty resided in me. And I wanted it to bubble up and spill over onto everyone I encountered, their own invitations into glory. Hers is the image in my mind when I say, "All bodies are good bodies." This shining, glorious freedom to encounter another with pure aliveness. My shadows were shame and fear about the size and enoughness of my body and my supposed lack of strong character to make myself smaller. I have tried to lean into the light of that pure-alive goodness, that liberation of my fat body. I follow the beacons left by the trailblazers ahead of me whose stories matter so much to me; it is an honor to share some of them with you.

In popular culture, we are told that the purpose of the human body is to be healthy. In popular Christian culture, we are told that the purpose of the human body is to serve others. But when we poke around even just a little bit at these concepts, we quickly learn that both "health" and "service" are coded words for thinness or trimness. We must examine how this concept of a good body as a healthy one ready to serve excludes people on the margins of society like those with disabilities, those with chronic illness, those who are old, and those who are very young. If health is our bodies' primary goal, achieving this goal becomes a Darwinian exercise in survival of the fittest. If service is our bodies' primary goal, achieving it becomes a kind of works-based salvation where young and abled bodies are privileged over aging and disabled ones.

No, the purpose of our bodies is neither thinness nor trimness, neither health nor service. The purpose of our bodies is relationship, with others and with ourselves and with God. This is the only purpose that brings everyone to the table, no matter the state of their health or the size of their body. I think the ancient Greek philosophers were on to something when they said that a thing is *good* if it fulfills its purpose. So, since bodies are made for the purpose of relationship, and people in any kind of bodies are capable of deep and meaningful relationships—bada bing, bada boom—all bodies are good bodies.

I can say this even as I look at my own body and see so many things that are considered not "good" about it: my fatness, my disability, my weakness, my mental illness, and my chronic pain, to name a few. However, I keep discovering that the most powerful thing is to bring my whole self to that table. My body is me and contains all my experiences, emotions, fears, pains, hopes, and dreams. My size cannot erase or restrict the beauty of all the friendship, romance, and adventure I've experienced in my nearly four decades on this planet. As I've learned to embrace my today body no matter what, I find that my capacity for connection expands to have relationships with other people who find themselves on the margins of our society.

As I enter the room and sit at the table in this fat body of mine, I am more than I have ever been before. I am flesh and bone, living cells of wonder, somehow made of water and dust and able to love. I contain within me the names and stories of the places I have been and the people I have met. I am full of contradictions and doubts and benedictions and truths. I do not have to make myself smaller to be lovable. My today body can hold all of this. My today body is enough, no matter what the others at the table think. All of this—all of me—is not too much. I don't need to be less than all of me; the world can just figure out how to handle more of me. And this isn't just body positivity in the way we think of it today. The term "body positivity" was originally used by people in marginalized fat bodies to describe their movement of body liberation and justice; today, body positivity denotes feeling good about one's body no matter the circumstance. It has been co-opted both by corporations (think Dove and its Real Beauty campaign) and by social media influencers (who exist in normal-sized bodies) to change our emotions and perceptions about our bodies without addressing the structural injustice that comes with being fat.

As a fat citizen in the United States, I have experienced exclusion, embarrassment, and harassment because of my body. Our country is literally not built to include me, and our laws are neither inclusive enough nor strong enough to protect my dignity. Yet there is light creeping up over the horizon. I can see that the cultural trajectory regarding bodies, health, and size is beginning to bend toward body justice, and that gives me hope. But there is a lot more work to be done, both in unlearning my internalized fat phobia and in educating others about how damaging fat phobia is for a child's well-being. If you want to make our culture a safer and more just place to exist in a fat body, as a fat citizen or as someone who loves a fat person, this book is for you.

As a person of Christian faith, I have struggled to reconcile this good body of mine with the untruths that persist within our halls of worship. I have questioned and shouted and made my displeasure known to a God whose people are supposed to be known by their love but who have pushed me away and called me names because of my body. I have fought to make places of worship more accepting and accessible, yet I still find that I am too big to fit in so many of those spaces, body and soul. If you have felt the same, this book is for you. This is a book about the relationship we have with our bodies and how that affects us, and how we can walk in the world around us and take up the space we deserve. I invite you to join me and all the other beautiful people on this journey. Together, we're building a bigger table with ample and sturdy seating. My sincere hope is that in these pages you find freedom and permission to love your body as it is today.

PACKING LIST

- **MY FAT IMAGINATION.** I actively employ my imagination so that I can envision who I want to be, where I want to go, or how I want to be treated. I can let my imagination run as wild as I want because I am the one making decisions for me. I've included the *who, what, where, how,* and *why* that exist in my fat imagination. It doesn't have to be in list form like mine is—you could make a vision board, make a painting, construct a PowerPoint presentation, or do a timeline in memes.

    WHAT I WANT TO EXPERIENCE: A world where every person is treated with dignity and compassion no matter their size, shape, ability, or level of health.

    WHO I WANT TO BE: Like the woman that C. S. Lewis describes in *The Great Divorce*, life and joy overflowing and spreading out around my fat body, spilling onto others.

WHERE I WANT TO GO: To a place where I am completely free to exist in my today body, where body size does not determine my worth or my level of access to public and private spaces.

HOW I WANT TO GET THERE: With a radical belief in the goodness of my body even with its weaknesses . . . even perhaps because of its weaknesses.

WHY I WANT TO GO THERE: To bring others along with me as we pursue peace and freedom so that we can change the world with our fat imaginations.

—— TOUCHSTONE ——

MY TODAY BODY IS GOOD.

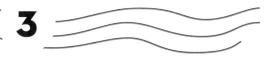

"FAT" IS NOT A BAD WORD

Fat: not a bad word; a morally neutral way to describe a body; an accessibility issue.

MY CHILDREN RECENTLY BEGGED TO WATCH the 1970 classic *Willy Wonka and the Chocolate Factory*, starring Gene Wilder. Even though Roald Dahl is one of my husband's favorite authors and Gene Wilder one of his favorite actors, I had resisted letting them watch it for years. Any good memories I have of watching the movie as a child are far outweighed by bad memories—even nightmarish ones. If you've seen the movie, you'll quickly recognize what I'm talking about.

In the film, five school-age children have won Golden Tickets to tour a secretive chocolate magnate's factory (in order of elimination along the tour): Augustus Gloop, Violet Beauregarde, Veruca Salt, Mike Teavee, and Charlie Bucket. To be honest, I saw the movie once decades ago, and I only remembered Charlie (because he was the protagonist) and the two characters who exemplify fatness in the film: Augustus Gloop and Violet Beauregarde.

Augustus is a very fat and impulsive child who disregards Wonka's warnings and contaminates the chocolate river when he falls in. He disappears under the water and is sucked up a tube, where he is stuck for a while before the pressure building up beneath him forcefully propels him along the tube and out of sight. His indiscretion is touching the pure chocolate stream, making it unclean. Never mind that everyone else is literally licking every other surface in the room; it's the fat kid who makes something unclean. When Augustus falls in, no one helps him. His mother, a portly woman herself, just stands there and yells at Willy Wonka to do something to help her son.

The feelings around fatness that this scene evoked in me? Guilt—if he hadn't been so greedy, he wouldn't have fallen in. It's his fault he's drowning in liquid chocolate. Helplessness—when you're fat and in trouble, no one is going to help you (possibly not even your parents). Stuckness—in the midst of this traumatic experience, Wonka and the others make fun of Augustus getting stuck in the tube; he is completely dehumanized and entirely objectified as a problem to be solved, not a person to be rescued. Watching a fat child on the screen endure this trauma marked me. I was afraid of getting stuck inside things because of my size, and this movie reinforced the fear and the possibility that no one would be able to help me or rescue me.

The other fat character is Violet Beauregarde, a champion bubblegum chewer who grabs one of Wonka's inventions—his newest bubblegum, of course—and begins to chew. It's a delicious three-course meal in one piece of candy! However, Violet ignores Wonka's mild warnings to stop chewing, and her impetuousness earns her the punishment of turning into a giant blueberry. The Oompa-Loompas roll her away to the juicing room, where she will be squeezed until all the juice is out of her so that she will not explode. What befell Violet echoed the fears I had about my body as a child. First of all, her body size was a punishment for what she ate. Second, she became a freak, and everyone commented about her body's changes. And, third, she had to be rolled away to a room where she would be made smaller.

There's no way my parents could have known that this film would become another voice in the chorus of fat phobia inside my head. But how I wish someone had talked with me after seeing that movie and said, "Amanda, they should have tried to help Augustus. It wasn't right that he was sucked up and stuck in that tube just because he ate the chocolate like everyone else. And what happened to Violet wasn't fair, even if she didn't listen to Mr. Wonka's warnings. When you bring kids into a tour of a candy factory, they should be safe, not dehumanized."

The reality is that we cannot shield our children from negative portrayals of fat people in the media they encounter. So what Zachary and I do with our four kids is watch TV with them and address negative fat stereotypes as they happen. The worst offender we have seen recently is in the Netflix original Christmas movie *Klaus* (2019). It's kind of a Hatfield-versus-McCoys story set in a snowy and remote village, where the young postmaster must make his post office successful to prove himself. Each of the feuding families has a very fat child among them, of very low intelligence and with almost no ability to communicate.

These characters were played strictly for laughs and to demonize the feuding families as the bad guys in the film.

When the movie ended, I asked our children (who at the time were seven, six, four, and two) these questions:

Did you notice any fat people in the movie?
How are they portrayed—good or bad, nice or evil,
simple or complex?
Do you know any fat people in real life?
Are they like the fat characters in the movie?
Are they different than the fat characters in the movie?

Because my kids are so young, they don't have complex answers for these questions. They mostly just answer yes or no at this point. But when we add these questions into the mix of all we are doing to promote the goodness of all bodies, I know they are learning to question the tropes and stereotypes that fat people are lazy, dumb, bumbling, and fit to be the butt of jokes. I make it a point to say the things I wish someone had said to me after my experience with Willy Wonka: *It's not okay for a person to be treated that way, no matter the size of their body. Someone's body size isn't a punishment. Body diversity is a beautiful thing. It's okay to be fat. There are all different kinds of fat people in the world, and they are all loved by God in their good bodies.*

We need to change the underlying meaning of fatness from dull, lazy, and monstrous to large size and moral neutrality. How do we do that? First, we must do the work internally, recognizing that fatness isn't a morality issue—it's an accessibility issue. At face value, fatness tells us nothing more about a body than does hair or eye color. Like my friend Valerie says, "Allow me to talk about myself using entirely morally neutral descriptors: female, short, brunette, blue-eyed, fat. Each of these descriptors serve to tell a person about my physical appearance. None of them says anything about who I am as a person. Our society has convinced us of a lot of things about what fat supposedly means, what fat people are like, and that fat is to be feared. I disagree."[1]

"FAT" IS NOT A BAD WORD

"Let me ask you a question," I projected. "When you see this body of mine, what three-letter f-word comes to mind?" It was one of the last rehearsals for a live storytelling, and I had written "Fitting In" about my experience as a bigger person born and bred in East Texas. I stood there in my size 30 dress with my knock knees, and when I finished rehearsing, one of the (male, in case that matters to you) acting consultants had a note for me: "Great job. I love your enthusiasm. But the three-letter f-word that came to my mind was 'fun,' not 'fat'!" His tone communicated more, implying that I didn't need to focus on my fatness because I was just so much fun! I smiled and explained that I'm okay with being fat, but today I would become the embodiment of the eye roll emoji and say, "It's okay to be fat."

Have you ever called yourself "fat" and had people be weird about it? It simultaneously amuses me and annoys me, being met with responses like "You're not fat; you're a lovely person" or "Fat isn't what our bodies *are*; it's something our bodies *have*." I recognize that people have been conditioned to recoil at fatness and that they are attempting to be kind to me. Their kindness comes in assuring me that they do not see me as a moral failure because of my body size. But people need to know that it's okay to be fat. And that means our understanding of the term needs to adapt.

Marilyn Wann says that we should use the word "fat" as a descriptor, not a discriminator.[2] The journey toward fully embracing fatness as a neutral descriptor was a slow one. I would call myself fat, but nobody else was allowed to. Even people who loved me and knew about my desire for body confidence couldn't. It still hurt too much because I had not become accustomed to hearing another person direct it at me in a nonthreatening way. I wanted to help others find freedom like I was doing, but "fat acceptance activist" was a burden to my ears. So I made up my own words; I became a "size-dignity activist." Yes, it was clunky, but it got a lot less pushback, both from my own psyche and from the people I thought I was trying to reach. When I finally tired of "size dignity" and had adjusted my view of the f-word internally, I embraced the word "fat" as all I needed. I am a fat activist. Whatever activism I do is as a fat person. And if you want to accept me as a person or as an activist, fatness is part of the Amanda Martinez Beck total package. I'm past managing others' emotions about how my self-descriptive language makes them feel.

Maybe you're fat; maybe you're not. Maybe you think you are or want to call yourself fat, but it's just too much for now. That's fine; I really do get that. But the tone of the word really has to shift. Because if it doesn't, it perpetuates our cultural hatred of fatness.

Language is a beloved and powerful tool. It can be simultaneously descriptive and prescriptive. It is descriptive in how it allows us to narrate and organize what we feel, think, observe, and believe. It is prescriptive in how we use it to call ourselves and others to a higher purpose and to encourage us along the way. We use the word "fat" in so many ways. Consider its uses below and identify if it is used neutrally, negatively, or positively.

> *"Ugh, I feel so fat today."*
> *"You earned a big fat zero on your assignment?"*
> *"I can't find anything to wear because I'm so fat."*
> *"If you weren't so fat, this wouldn't have happened."*
> *"You're so fat!"*
> *"Because I'm fat, I need access to alternative seating, please."*

These statements offer various ways that we perceive fatness in our society. Let's take a look at how "fat" is used in each of these scenarios.

1. *"Ugh, I feel so fat today."*
   The tone here is negative, referring to the speaker's discomfort with their body. This feeling of discomfort and frustration may be caused by bloating or tiredness upon physical exertion. It's okay to feel discomfort in your body. However, we must make clear that *fatness is not a feeling*; it's a state of a person's body size that cannot change perceptively from one day to another. *Feeling* deals with emotion. *Fat* deals with size.

2. *"You earned a big fat zero on your assignment?"*
   The tone here is negative, with the word "fat" used as
   a negative intensifier. It communicates that receiving a
   zero on an assignment is unquestionably bad. If I hear
   this; I will point out that *fatness is not a negative state of
   being;* it is a neutral descriptor of size, and I'll want to see
   the actual zero on the paper to verify if it is indeed drawn
   very large. When my kids use the phrase "big fat," I tell
   them it's to be used positively or neutrally, and we don't
   use it toward other people unless that is what they ask us
   to call them. I tend to avoid using it. However, if everyone
   in the donut shop has a small little hoop of fried dough
   but the lady gives me one three times the normal size,
   I'll positively say, "Now, *that's* a big fat donut!" And I'll be
   glad and right. See also: "Now, *that's* a big fat paycheck!"
   if I am handed a large royalty check for this book in the
   future and "I would like that big fat piece of bacon right
   there" if I am staying at a fancy hotel with a sit-down
   breakfast.

3. *"I can't find anything to wear because I'm so fat."*
   This statement can have two distinct meanings in our
   cultural landscape. For people in thinner bodies, whose
   clothing sizes fall between women's sizes 00 and 12 and
   men's waist sizes up to 36 (often referred to as "straight
   sizes"), a statement like this is simply not true and is
   therefore not the correct usage of "fat." If clothes their
   size are out of stock in one store, it is easy and practical
   for someone in straight sizing to go to another store
   nearby to shop. However, when the person saying

"I can't find anything to wear because I'm fat" lives in a larger body (i.e., sizes 14 and up), it is most often true in a literal sense. Plus-size clothing options are limited in most stores, and we are forced to find professional, fashionable, and even practical clothing on the internet. Which, I'll tell you, is a big game of hit or miss. For the love of the girls, I can't tell you how much I would give for a bra that actually fits! Being able to try on such an undergarment is a luxury fat people aren't often afforded.

4. *"If you weren't so fat, this wouldn't have happened."*
I recognize this from my own feelings of shame. It has lived rent-free in my head more often than I'd like to admit. It's also a pretty convenient blame game when a fat person experiences an injury or an illness. I've heard doctors use it for everything from broken elbows to infertility to stomach cancer. What the literal frack? Fatness *can* be something that someone chooses to be. But, also, we don't really understand as much as we think we do about weight and health and body size or shape. A lot of body stuff we claim to have control over is actually genetic. And many other factors, like access to food and health care and the privilege of exercise, are beyond individual choice. We've got to stop blaming individuals for body issues and instead help change the system that perpetuates injustice.

5. *"You're so fat!"*
Fat as an insult: I don't think this one needs much explanation. When people try to use fatness as the butt

of a joke, I see it for the laziness it is. Body size is neutral and boring. Seriously, bro—is that the best you can do? Thank you . . . next!

6. *"Because I'm fat, I need access to alternative seating, please."*
Ah, finally a neutral use. A descriptor of a body's size, not an insult or judgment or mask to hide behind.

To change how we feel about fatness, we have to change how we talk about fatness. If it is truly neutral (which it is, because body size is morally neutral), we can use the word "fat" interchangeably with other adjectives we claim about ourselves, like brunette or brown-eyed or short. We can challenge when it is used as shorthand for bad character traits, and we can make sure to fill our lives and our stories with narratives of fat, happy, good, and joyful people.

FATNESS IS AN ACCESSIBILITY ISSUE

If fatness is not a feeling, a moral issue, a negative amplifier, or an insult, then what is it? It's a neutral descriptor of a large body that often faces personal and systemic prejudice and exclusion. My friend J. Nicole Morgan taught me an easy way to judge if your body *is* fat rather than just feeling fat: the chair test. Ask yourself this question: When I go into a new place, do I need to be concerned with whether the available seating will accommodate my body? If so, that is a sign that you are probably what I mean by "fat." Another question you can ask yourself is "Do I find clothes at typical clothing stores, or must I shop at specialty stores?" Fat people often do not have the ability to walk into Target and find something to their tastes that fits; if they are able to find clothing in their sizes, there is often only one style, no choices.

Another way to frame the concept of fatness is accessibility. In a fat body, many things are difficult to access, from clothing and adequate health care to public spaces and transportation. You can ask yourself to what extent your daily experience is limited or restricted by the size of your body. When I was in college and thought I was fat, I faced medical fat phobia and internalized fat phobia. However, I was still able to travel with no problem and move in public and private areas without concern of having enough space for my body. My body has grown and changed since that time (because bodies are meant to change as we age), and now I do have to consider seating options and clothing availability wherever I go, as well as fight for compassionate medical care and guard against unjust discrimination due to my size.

When we consider fatness as an accessibility issue, it opens up other useful discourses. For example, can fatness be classified as a disability? There is a lot of overlap between fat liberation and disability activism, such as advocating for the dignity of every human body, appropriate medical care, and elimination of discrimination based on the body; pushing against the infantilization of the body; and recognizing the agency of every person no matter the state of their body. On one hand, classifying fatness as a disability could give legal protection from discrimination under the Americans with Disabilities Act (ADA). Fat people could benefit from a law ensuring that their employers must accommodate them. At my last job, the building was built before the ADA was passed, and there were no handicap bathroom stalls. This is an accessibility issue that the ADA covers. Using the bathroom was a daily issue; I had to travel two floors down to find the one bathroom in the building that had the one stall that I could access without pain. I did advocate for myself and ask for accommodations to be made, and though I was assured that they would rectify the situation, nothing ever changed.

On the other hand, because of the harmful ways our society views people living with disabilities (a topic that could fill another entire book), identifying fatness as a disability could intensify the existing cultural attitude of fatness as a liability rather than as an asset. As I live in a fat and disabled body, I experience this on the reg. Just check out my Facebook author page. The photo of me wearing my "All Bodies Are Good Bodies" t-shirt *and* my oxygen cannula a few weeks after getting discharged from my COVID-19 hospital stay? I have deleted so many comments from people ridiculing me not just for my size but also my oxygen dependence. Fatness and disability are equally negative in the minds of so many people I encounter. Well, fatness is always considered the worse of the two if they are paired together because, I am told, my fatness has caused all my health problems. As if people in thin- or average-sized bodies never get sick or become disabled. Insert double eye-roll emoji.

Changing the tone and context around the concepts of fatness and disability is an important part of the work. Pressing for fat accessibility is too.

PACKING LIST

Challenging fat stereotypes:

- In media portrayals, ask:
  - Did you notice any fat people in the movie?
  - How are they portrayed: good or bad, nice or evil, simple or complex?
  - Do you know any fat people in real life?
  - Are they like the fat characters in the movie?
  - Are they different than the fat characters in the movie?
- In negative language, ask:
  - How can I communicate my feelings and needs without denigrating fatness?
  - Do I make fatness the butt of jokes, even self-deprecating ones?
- In terms of accessibility, ask:
  - Are the places I frequent (work, restaurants, stores, places of worship, etc.) friendly to fat bodies?
  - How can I use my voice to advocate for fat bodies?
    - Ask for inclusive seating with armless and sturdy seats.
    - Ask for sizes larger than my own to be stocked.

─── **TOUCHSTONE** ───

"FAT" IS NOT A BAD WORD.

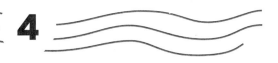

4

IT'S OKAY TO BE FAT

Fat liberation: a freedom movement, birthed in the 1960s, emphasizing natural body diversity and embracing fatness and the right of fat people to dignified treatment in every area of life. Fat liberation tears down systemic fat oppression at every level: personal, interpersonal, community-based, and structural. It addresses the need for and the obstacles against the inclusion of fat people and creates a world where it truly is okay to be fat.

IT'S OKAY TO BE FAT. When I communicate this—no matter how eloquently or bluntly—it brings my fat-phobic followers out of the woodwork. Mind you, I'm normally just saying it's okay to be fat, not that everyone should be fat or that being thin is wrong. But people feel personally attacked as if I have said those things. Fat = bad is so ingrained in us. But no matter what the trolls, your inner self-critic, or your parents say, it's okay to be fat, and being fat is okay. Now more than ever, we must proclaim this truth, not just from fat mouths but from mouths of all sizes. Honestly, it feels like a brave thing to say, even though it shouldn't be a question. There is nothing wrong with being fat, precisely because body size is morally neutral. It's okay to be whatever size you are because body size does not indicate whether you're a good or bad person. Let me repeat: body size is morally neutral; body size does not indicate whether you're a good or bad person. Bodies, regardless of size, are both very good and very neutral—good because they enable us to really be *us* and to have relationships with God and other humans and the whole universe. Neutral insofar as one body is worth as much as any other body, worthy of dignified treatment and compassion. Our thin-obsessed culture treats body worthiness as a zero-sum game—that is, that there is only so much "goodness" of bodies to go around, so some people will have a lot, and some people will have none. But the truth is that goodness—which comes from the image of God within us—is an unlimited resource.

Health status is morally neutral too, so if someone needs it to be stated clearly, here it is: Physical health is not the end-all of life, neither is it a noble moral good. Fatness does not equal lack of health, but even if it did, it would still be okay to be fat. We do not owe health to anyone—not our moms or our spouses or our children, and definitely not to strangers! This kind of thinking excludes people in chronically ill and disabled bodies, and it's a hallmark of ableism.

When I say it's okay to be fat, I mean that it is also okay to *look* fat. But too often, people in fat bodies are asked to hide or obscure their bodies for the comfort of others. Fashion is an area where fat bodies have not only been ignored but intentionally excluded. In 2016, fashion guru Tim Gunn wrote an excoriating opinion piece for the *Washington Post* decrying the entrenched fat phobia in his industry. The title gives the thesis of the piece: "Designers refuse to make clothes to fit American women. It's a disgrace."[1] Gunn goes on to say,

> I love the American fashion industry, but it has a lot of problems, and one of them is the baffling way it has turned its back on plus-size women. It's a puzzling conundrum. The average American woman now wears between a size 16 and a size 18, according to new research from Washington State University. There are 100 million plus-size women in America, and for the past three years, they have increased their spending on clothes faster than their straight-size counterparts. There is money to be made here ($20.4 billion, up 17 percent from 2013). But many designers—dripping with disdain, lacking imagination or simply too cowardly to take a risk—still refuse to make clothes for them.

Gunn himself reveals his own fat phobia in his article, encouraging designers to employ slimming techniques to create optical illusions. "Done right, our clothing can create an optical illusion that helps us look taller and slimmer. Done wrong, and we look worse than if we were naked." Tim, honey, I'm all for cool design, but I want be perceived as I actually am, how I live and move and have my being in this world. I'm enough. I'm not too much. I don't need to appear taller or slimmer to be my full, attractive, abundant self. I don't owe thinness to anyone, so it follows that I'm not obligated to "trick" anyone into believing that part of me is not actually there. Honestly, that's silly. Even if I'm wearing all black or vertical stripes (or both), it's still very obvious that I am a fat woman. I do not have to diminish myself for the sake of pleasing others.

When Gunn's article came out, I was conflicted. On the one hand, I was so glad that the fashion industry was being called to account for its fat phobia by one of its biggest names. On the other hand, I could still see the blatant fat phobia within the article itself, which was disheartening. How could Tim Gunn be so right while still being so wrong? I had to learn a way to rescue the good while letting go of the rest, a skill that comes in very useful as I see the journey toward fat acceptance and body liberation of people I know and people in the national spotlight.

A NARROW HISTORY OF A WIDE SUBJECT

When I first encountered the radical idea of fat liberation, my curiosity pushed me to learn where it began. It was a relief to realize that there was an army of fat activists doing the hard work long before I was even born. As far as I am able to discern, the American fat liberation movement began with a twentysomething Jewish man, Steve Post, just getting his start in the New York radio scene. (As I share the stories of fat liberation ahead, please know that mine is a narrow approach to a wide subject; it would be remiss not to warn you that this is not the whole story of fat liberation. Disabled, fat, and queer activists have done so much of the brain and legwork to get us to where we are today. The history of fat liberation that I weave into my chapters is very much only part of the story; please see the recommended readings for more detail.)

In 1967, Steve Post organized the first-ever Fat-In in New York City. Steve had grown up in the '40s and '50s with "extra" weight. As he matured, his body slimmed down. But here's the kicker—he missed his formerly bigger and heavier body. (So countercultural, right?) He observed how the prevailing attitude about bodies in his time celebrated—and even championed—thinness as the ideal, popularized by many celebrities including Twiggy, a supermodel with a name descriptive of her body. The year 1967 was a year of cultural unrest; people were protesting the war in Vietnam, and it was the summer of drugs, sex, and rock and roll at Woodstock. So Steve Post decided to protest. To do so, he gathered approximately five hundred people in Sheep Meadow of New York City's Central Park on June 4.

The next day, a small unattributed article appeared on page 54L of the *New York Times*, next to a large ad for "Top Broadway Hits." The article was titled "Curves Have Their Day in the Park; 500 at a Fat-In Call for Obesity." According to the article, Post claimed that fat people were discriminated against, saying, "The advertising campaigns have attempted to make us feel guilty about our size . . . People should be proud of being fat. We want to show we feel happy, not guilty. That's why we're here." Among the five hundred protestors gathered for the fat-in, people held signs that said things like "Fat Power" and carried food in their hands, as they had been encouraged to do. Some burned diet books, and others burned images of Twiggy. (That is unfortunate; no one deserves to be burned in effigy.) Though Post's fat liberation activism seems to have faded after the fat-in, the protest was a catalyst that spurred the fat liberation movement forward. Post would go on to establish himself as a pillar in the radio industry, but any other fat liberation work he may have done has been lost to posterity.

A few months after the fat-in, the *Saturday Evening Post* published an article by the writer Lew Louderback called "More People Should Be Fat." It made its way to homes across the United States in the November 4, 1967, issue. Louderback lamented the way that fat people were treated, asserting, "There's something distinctly unhealthy, even sinister, in the anti-fat madness that has swept this country in recent years." He goes on to recount how America's obsession with thinness, what he calls "the slimness cult," has led to repeated violations against fat people's civil rights: fat employees who have lost their jobs after failing to meet company-directed weight-loss standards and college applicants turned down because of their body sizes. He also noted that the foods considered healthy were more expensive than simple starches, making it costlier to eat "better."

Louderback explained that, for a long time, he and his wife—whom he describes as "naturally fat"—devoted themselves to dieting, but their slim phases never lasted more than six months at a time. In a striking parallel to my own story, they finally decided to escape the never-ending demands of the slimness cult, and they made peace with their bodies. He describes their experience after quitting "thin culture" like this: "Each pound that we put on made us feel physically better, more relaxed. We discovered that we could finally concentrate on what we were doing. No longer did we live with one eye on the refrigerator, the other on the clock. Food lost its importance. As a matter of fact, we rarely thought about it."

Louderback confessed that at first, he and his wife were concerned about their health. However, their research in that area yielded surprising information about fatness. For example, he wrote of finding evidence that showed that weight fluctuation caused by dieting could be very dangerous, and in the event of a heart attack, fat patients had a greater chance of surviving than thin ones. (Sadly, he didn't cite which source he got this from, but y'all, this was in or before 1967!) He even noted that women who had a positive attitude toward food and eating were more sexually responsive. The article touches on the effects of class, career, education, giving yourself full permission to eat, the natural-weight plateau, "what about health?" challenges, science revealing that diets don't work, harmful beauty ideals, representation, and a call to "follow the money"—in under twenty-five hundred words. All of which are current topics of discussion in the modern fat liberation community.

He concluded his article with the hope that the culture around him would come to see the dangers of the slimness cult and make space for fat people to live their lives in peace, without discrimination. Louderback's article got him a book deal for *Fat Power*, but the book released to a critically negative audience. The small publisher with which he originally contracted was bought by Hawthorn Books mid-writing, which meant the loss of the editor championing Lew. Somehow the book went to print without Louderback's bibliography of research references. Suffice it to say that with the negative pushback and lack of research references provided to back up his revolutionary proto-fat-liberation "fat-power" position, Louderback's book failed to reach people who needed to read his message. It's no surprise that *Fat Power* is out of print now, a half century after its publication, and extant copies are quite near impossible to be found.

BILL FABREY AND NAAFA

Bill Fabrey grew up as a thin kid but, as a teenager, discovered—in his words—that he was a fat admirer, meaning that he was attracted to women of size. Fabrey felt alone as a fat admirer, but Lew Louderback's *Saturday Evening Post* article caught his eye. Three years earlier, Fabrey had married Joyce, a fat woman, and he observed how poorly others treated her because of her body size. He remembers when they applied for a marriage certification. It was 1964, and New York State law required a blood test as part of the effort to stop the spread of syphilis.[2] When Joyce went to the test to get her blood drawn, Fabrey relates that the doctor "asked why she was there . . . Joyce replied that she was engaged to be married soon and needed to obtain a blood test. The astonished doctor replied, 'Who would want to marry you?'"

Fabrey reached out to Louderback, and soon Bill and Joyce found themselves helping Lew and his wife with research for *Fat Power*. Even though Joyce was less than convinced by the data on fatness and health, discussion among them lead to an idea: they could create a mutual support for people in the fat community. That's when they decided to found the National Association to Aid Fat Americans (NAAFA). The NAAFA constitution was signed and ratified by the founding members on June 13, 1969.

Fabrey says early meetings were very awkward, with little eye contact and a lot of suspicion, but that's understandable. When you're labeled and treated as a social pariah, it takes time to build trust. Finding hospitality when you're used to hostility can be a shock to your system.

To boost attendance, they needed something more attractive (literally): NAAFA dating. Due to this addition and a growing interest in fat acceptance, NAAFA exploded from New York City to the West Coast. However, as NAAFA meetings became more about socializing and finding romance, many leaders (including Louderback) withdrew from the organization. They believed that activism and accompanying education were the conduits of societal challenge of fat phobia and embracing of fat liberation. Eventually, however, the leaders of NAAFA changed its name to the National Association to Advance Fat Acceptance to reflect a more explicit mission of liberation. It is still a vanguard in fat activism today, crafting policy and combatting fat phobia through education and legal avenues, helping to create a world where it is okay to be fat.

LIBERATING THE OPPRESSED

I have to be honest with you, reader. There is much in this early history of fat liberation that does not sit well with me. Bill Fabrey's "fat admirer" concept borders on fetishization to me, and I am angry that Steve Post seemingly abandoned the public work of fat liberation after the fat-in. I'm disappointed that Lew Louderback did not save the bibliographical evidence for *Fat Power* and that his publisher was so hostile to the project. Also, in a world of intersectionality, where the oppressed are more often than not the custodians of wisdom, I wish there was more written about the early contributions to fat liberation by women, by fat BIPOC (Black, Indigenous, people of color), and by LGBTQIA+ fat folk.

So, on this journey, we won't find a flawless, justice-oriented, inclusive pedigree of fat liberation thought and theory. Parts of this story will be too much for us to process in one sitting, or too liberal or conservative or radical or pedestrian for our view of the world. Like Tim Gunn's article and his fat-phobic callout of the fashion industry's anti-fat bias, we confront the flaws while we celebrate the truths, the nuggets of wisdom along the way. We get to practice holding on to the treasures that truly liberate us while rejecting what oppresses us. And I'm including myself in this litmus test too—if some of the things I'm saying sounds like freedom and others feel threatening, take what brings you peace and chuck the rest. The road is long and wearisome, but remember—you're not alone on this journey, and together we are making a world where it is okay to be fat.

PACKING LIST

- Liberating the oppressed: how to do this for yourself and others to create a world where it is okay to be fat. Examine the narratives and history around you. Ask yourself:
  - What about this narrative needs to be different in order to be truly just? What gems of wisdom are here?

- How does this change my life?
- How does this bring freedom to oppressed people?
- With whom do I need to share this?

TOUCHSTONE

IT'S OKAY TO BE FAT.

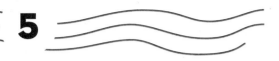

5

YOU HAVE THE RIGHT TO TAKE UP SPACE

Politics: what happens when bodies take up space near each other, the fallout from this, and its organization.

BODIES ARE INHERENTLY POLITICAL. Mind you, I'm not talking partisanship; there are no inherently Republican or Democratic bodies. My definition of politics is what happens when bodies take up space near each other. And if you can believe it, I have been told I was a communist liberal for suggesting that a person may take up the space they need with the body they're in. I have been called all sorts of names for saying this. I have been subjected to the ugliest threats against my own body and against my marriage and my family. You know why? I think it might have to do with what Lynn Mabel-Lois and Sara Aldebaran say in the essay "Fat Women and Women's Fear of Fat": "Fear of fat is a means of social control used against all women. The current ideal woman's body is so thin that many women with quite average figures consider themselves to be too fat. A woman is warned that if she 'lets herself go,' her husband will leave her, she will have no lovers, and she will be miserable."[1]

To imply that a person—particularly a woman—has the right to take up as much space as she needs flies in the face of patriarchal social constructs that keep women smaller and quieter than their nature and biology incline them to be. I grew up in Southern Evangelical culture, where I took to heart the virtues of demureness and soft speaking. If you know me now, that's for sure not who I am! Letting my body and my soul take up all the space they need has made me a force to be reckoned with. Sometimes bringing my full self into a situation creates room for more people to do the same. Sometimes it leads to others feeling threatened. Most times, it's a combination of both. The same thing happened to the early pioneers of the fat liberation movement.

RADICAL, FEMINIST, AND FAT

In our tour of fat liberation history that began in the last chapter, we left off after Bill Fabrey and Lew Louderback founded NAAFA. As NAAFA expanded (pun always intended) with chapters on the East and West Coasts, divisions within the burgeoning fat liberation community began to reveal themselves. In her landmark book *Fat Activism: Radical Social Movement*, fat academic Charlotte Cooper writes, "NAAFA's public face was one of social action, but the organization also functioned as a meeting place for fat women and [the] men who were sexually attracted to them."[2] In a 2008 email to Cooper, Bill Fabrey himself acknowledged that one of his motivations in cofounding NAAFA was to normalize being a fat admirer: "I wanted to make the world a safer and more pleasant place for persons of size, and for them to like themselves better, and lastly, and less important, for nobody to tell me what my taste should be."[3]

I admit that this quote makes me squirm quite a bit. It feels disingenuous not to acknowledge that this kind of thinking is only a few steps away from fetishizing fatness and justifying it from a male-centered perspective, also called the male gaze. Fat people should be free to exist with confidence without being objectified because of their sizes. Indeed, as women's liberation progressed in the United States, Fabrey's fat admiration approach, centering the heterosexual male gaze, alienated many fat women involved with NAAFA. From the stories I've read, many male NAAFA attendees have assumed that fat women are desperate for any male attention they can get, which of course breeds an environment of harassment and assault.

Many members prioritized fat social activism and discrimination over fat socializing. Fat activist Vivian Mayer recounts, "The fat women's liberation movement in Los Angles grew out of the blending of two sources, radical feminism and radical therapy."[4] According to Mayer, in the 1970s, traditional therapy convinced the patient that the problem lies in themselves, asking them to change themselves to accommodate an unjust and oppressive world. Radical therapy, on the other hand, resounded with a well-known feminist slogan: "the personal is political." Instead of demanding that fat bodies become smaller to fit into an unjust world, radical therapy gives a framework in which fat people possess the power to insist that the unjust world must change. As a fat woman in my thirties, I am so thankful for this way of seeing my fatness—when the culture rejects me for my body size, it's the culture that must change, not my body.

Fat Jewish feminists Judy Freespirit (also known as Vivian F. Mayer) and Aldebaran (also known as Sara Golda Bracha Fishman) used radical feminist therapy to expose the cultural mechanisms that oppressed fat women, especially within medicine. Along with medical research librarian Lynn Mabel-Lois (later Lynn McAfee), Freespirit and Aldebaran formed their own NAAFA chapter in Los Angeles. They were serious about challenging the world's anti-fat bias within medicine, and when NAAFA shied away from this task, these women had to cut ties with Bill Fabrey's organization.

Fat Underground

Although Freespirit, Aldebaran, and McAfee were not the only ones to splinter off from NAAFA and form their own activism-heavy group (pun always intended), these women founded the most well-known one: Fat Underground. Using the framework they had encountered through radical feminist therapy, Freespirit and Aldebaran wrote the *Fat Liberation Manifesto*, a seven-point document stating the dignity of fat people, their anger at the exploitation of fat people commercially and sexually, how their oppression is related to other forms of oppression in our society, an explicit rejection of diet culture and its pseudoscientific claims, and their refusal to surrender their power to their enemies. The manifesto ends with this lien in all caps: "FAT PEOPLE OF THE WORLD, UNITE! YOU HAVE NOTHING TO LOSE. . . ."[5]

Heavy Changes

"It's important for fat women to understand that you're gonna have to go through some really heavy changes, and that things that were told to you, things that you grew up believing, are lies on a really deep level, on a really painful level." I stared at my computer, watching a fuzzy black-and-white picture moving in front of me. A super-fat woman is sitting on a living room chair, sitting like I do sometimes—knees out on either side of the chair. The audio quality was terrible, but I had to hear more.

"It's very easy to just dismiss what's being said—'Oh, *they're* just people who couldn't diet successfully.' We've all dieted successfully many times and have all gotten fatter. And we have statistics to back us up, if that's important to you. What should be more important to you is *your* experience, the fact that *you* have dieted many times and gained it back. The fact that you have to live through tomorrow when you have to try and get into your bathing suit."

Her words stung a little, but I heard what she was telling me. Her name is Lynn McAfee, and though she said all this (and more) in the late 1970s, she was speaking to me, a person who didn't even exist when she recorded this. This video was salvaged, along with a few other clips, all in all totaling about thirty-five minutes of film. That's all the film left of the Fat Underground, which makes me angry, because I want more. More witness to the reality of fat living before I was born, more fat women speaking clearly and powerfully about the dangers of dieting. More calling out the complicity of members of the medical profession in perpetuating harm against fat humans. More of *me*.

The women of the Fat Underground did more than record themselves for posterity. Members protested weight-loss clinics and gave lectures on the dangers of dieting. When fat woman and world-renowned singer "Mama" Cass Elliot, of the Mamas and the Papas, died at only thirty-two years old, people were quick to blame it on Cass's fatness. It was her physician, Anthony Greenburg, who speculated (before the autopsy) that she died eating a ham sandwich while lying in bed. However, an autopsy revealed that there was nothing in her throat, but the left side of her heart was extremely weak. At the time, the ham sandwich rumor spread like wildfire, and the abhorrent references to "Mama Cass's sandwich" still abound in pop culture. But the women of the Fat Underground knew that Cass had been dieting, and they suspected her death was hastened because of it.[6] According to the coroner's report, she died of a heart attack in her sleep, without food in her stomach and no drugs in her system. A few weeks after her death on July 29, 1974, the Women's Equality Day celebration in Los Angeles had an open mic on a large stage. The following is Aldebaran's memory of that day: "We carried candles and wore black arm bands, in a symbolic funeral procession. Lynn [McAfee] spoke. She began by describing the inspiration Cass Elliot had represented to us, as a fat woman who had refused to hide her beauty. She ended by accusing the medical establishment of murdering Cass, and (because they promote weight loss despite its known dangers) of committing genocide against fat women."[7]

The group enjoyed local fame for a while, but internal divisions in the radical feminist therapy movement caused many Fat Underground members to leave Los Angeles. The remaining members carried on their fat liberation work for a few years, but numbers dwindled. Powerful but short-lived, the Fat Underground became defunct in 1983 with the death of its last member, Reanna Fagan.[8]

From the late '70s into the early '80s, many former members of the Fat Underground, dispersed around the country, continued the work of fat liberation. Judy Freespirit and fellow fat liberationist Sharon Bas Hannah wrote and gathered writings about the cause. When no publisher would take on their *Shadow on a Tightrope* book, they took it upon themselves to print and distribute their work under the name Fat Liberation Press. It included the *Fat Liberation Manifesto*, which is printed below in its entirety:

THE FAT LIBERATION MANIFESTO

1. We believe that fat people are fully entitled to human respect and recognition.
2. We are angry at mistreatment by commercial and sexist interests. These have exploited our bodies as objects of ridicule, thereby creating an immensely profitable market selling the false promise of avoidance of, or relief from, that ridicule.
3. We see our struggle as allied with the struggles of other oppressed groups, against classism, racism, sexism, ageism, capitalism, imperialism, and the like.
4. We demand equal rights for fat people in all aspects of life, as promised in the Constitution of the United States. We demand equal access to goods and services in the public domain, and an end to discrimination against us in

the areas of employment, education, public facilities and health services.

5. We single out as our special enemies the so called "reducing" industries. These include diet clubs, reducing salons, fat farms, diet doctors, diet books, diet foods and food supplements, surgical procedures, appetite suppressants, drugs and gadgetry such as wraps and "reducing machines." We demand that they take responsibility for their false claims, acknowledge that their products are harmful to the public health, and publish long-term studies proving any statistical efficacy of their products. We make this demand knowing that over 99% of all weight loss programs, when evaluated over a 5-year period, fail utterly, and also knowing the extreme, proven harmfulness of repeated large changes in weight.

6. We repudiate the mystified "science" which falsely claims that we are unfit. It as both caused and upheld discrimination against us, in collusion with the financial interests of insurance companies, the fashion and garment industries, reducing industries, the food and drug establishments.

7. We refuse to be subjected to the interests of our enemies. We fully intend to reclaim power over our bodies and lives. We commit ourselves to pursue these goals together.

FAT PEOPLE OF THE WORLD, UNITE!
YOU HAVE NOTHING TO LOSE.

—Judy Freespirit and Aldebaran, November 1973[9]

Look at the date the manifesto was published. Half a century ago, and yet we are still fighting the same battles. The words are powerful and haunting because so little has changed. I believe that, as a society, we are in desperate need to realize the first point of the manifesto: "We believe that fat people are fully entitled to human respect and recognition." Modern treatment of fat people is despicable, ranging from ignoring them as if they don't exist to vilifying a fat person's character and mere existence.

In the vein of points one and four of the manifesto—the dignity of the fat person and the rights guaranteed by the US Constitution for fat people—I have developed a tool called The Fat Girl's Bill of Rights.

THE FAT GIRL'S BILL OF RIGHTS

1. **I have the right to exist in my today body.** My body's size neither diminishes my humanity nor my value in this world. Body size is morally neutral. The size of my body does not indicate the kind of person I choose to be or the work ethic that I have. My body is good (Genesis 2). When God finished making all of creation, God leaned back and looked and said it was good. But when God created humans, God said—even more emphatically—that it was *very* good. I want to live my life in that goodness, enjoying the world around me and trusting that the goodness of my body is because I am created in the image of a good God and that God has made me for relationship with God, with myself, and with others.

2. **I have the right to take up the space that I need.** I do not have to make myself smaller to accommodate the people around me because I have just as much right to live and move freely in this world as any person. I will advocate for myself to be given the space that I need to live and move and be free. God gives me an abundant life (John 10:10). One thing that living in a fat body has taught me is that the abundant life is a tangible reality. God isn't asking me to make myself smaller and take up less space. In fact, Hebrew scriptures speak of taking up even *more* space as a good thing (Isaiah 54:2).

3. **I have the right to eat the foods that I want to eat.** No one may tell me what I can or cannot eat based on my body size. Diets don't work for most people, and they mess with the body in ways we are only beginning to discover. Food freedom is the best approach for a thriving and peaceful relationship with food and my body. Consider Peter's vision in Acts 10. There is no such thing as an unclean food when we are speaking about the morality of eating. No group of nutrients is less okay for me to eat than any other, and no one has the right to shame me for my food choices. When we think about food as clean and unclean, it inevitably impacts how we think about the people who eat these foods.

4. **I have the right to wear whatever I want.** I reject the cultural rules of what a fat person can or cannot wear. I will wear what I consider appropriate for each situation I am in. I will advocate for more inclusivity in the fashion industry to make clothing for fat people more accessible. I do not give anyone permission to tell me how I need to

dress my fat body. It is for freedom that Christ has set me free, y'all—not to follow arbitrary clothing rules (Galatians 5:1). Fat girls shouldn't have a different dress code than other women just because we're fat. Everyone should have the right to wear the clothes they feel best in.

5. **I have the right to compassionate and informed fat-aware medical care.** I refuse to be treated without the same respect and autonomy as a person in a socially acceptable body. I recognize my right to refuse to be weighed at the doctor's office and my right to demand peer-reviewed studies and evidence for the medical advice given to me by my health-care provider. I refuse to receive any diagnosis without the proper medical testing, and I will refuse to discuss my weight with my doctor if I so desire. I have the right to medical care from a provider without defending myself from queries about stomach amputation (commonly known as weight-loss surgery). James 2 teaches us that there is no partiality with God, but that is not something I have seen reflected in the Christian doctors' offices that I have been to. If there are different standards of care and attention for people of different sizes, that's favoritism, and that's something that the Bible condemns. So even if you believe that fat people are less deserving of thorough medical care than thin people, it's wrong to treat us differently. In fact, if you read Matthew 25, it's pretty clear that the way you treat fat people matters to Jesus, because he identifies himself with those on the margins of society like sick people and prisoners.

6. **I have the right to maintain my boundaries over my body.** No one has the right to touch me without my

permission, and no one has the right to comment on my body. When I experience fat phobia, I have the right to speak the truth about body size and weight stigma. In addition to being able to put up boundaries about how people can talk to us about our bodies, fat girls also have the right to turn down someone who is interested in them romantically without being threatened. Our culture tells us that we should be thankful for any romance if we are fat, so it can feel intimidating to say no. Maybe we won't be asked out again. Maybe we will seem ungrateful. But it is very important that we know our freedom to say yes or no and have that be honored (Matthew 5:37).

7. **I have the right to move my body in any way I choose.** This extends to exercising without fat shaming and without being anyone's inspiration. I do not give permission for anyone to approach me in a gym or other context to give me unsolicited advice about my body or the exercise I am enjoying. I have the right to move freely about the gym and take up the space that my body needs. I do not have to defer to the desires of the culturally acceptable bodies in the gym or give them preference to workout machines or other limited gym resources. I don't think Moses's sister Miriam got permission from anyone when she started singing and dancing after God parted the Red Sea (Exodus 15:20).

8. **I have the right to live a public life without ridicule or abuse because of my body.** I have the right to live without the fearmongering of fat phobia. When interacting in public and private spaces, I do not have to listen to others threaten me with premature death,

loneliness, or cultural rejection based on the size of my body. I know that people in fat bodies can live long, happy lives with their loved ones. It's wrong to make fun of someone for their body. Some folks think that fat jokes and criticism of fat bodies are okay because they can motivate people to change. However, shame is a horrible motivator, so their argument is null. And, anyway, God operates not through shame but through kindness (Jeremiah 31:3).

9. **I have the right to reject diet culture.** I do not owe thinness or health to anyone. I can make whatever choices I desire about what I eat and how I move, whether I want to attempt weight loss or lean into the goodness of my body as it is today. I do not have to pursue intentional weight loss or try to make myself smaller. Dietary rules are of no benefit to my spiritual life (Colossians 2:16–23).

10. **I have the right to embrace the mystery of my body.** I am free to enjoy my today body just as it is, with all its complexity and mystery, without needing to control every aspect of its function and appearance. I can believe that my today body is not too much and that my today body is enough. My body isn't a machine that demands fuel; my body is me, and all of me is worthy of awe.

As fat people learn to claim these rights and live them out, the world will change. It starts small, one rock skipped across the waters of the status quo, with small ripples. But as more of us lean into these rights, a million little stones can cause a tidal wave so big that it will change the landscape for the better.

PACKING LIST

THE FAT GIRL'S BILL OF RIGHTS: Try standing in front of a mirror and speaking these rights to yourself in the first person. You may experience some internal resistance at first but repeat them over and over again until they feel true and deeply rooted in your soul.

1. I have the right to exist in my body today.
2. I have the right to take up space.
3. I have the right to eat the foods I want to eat.
4. I have the right to wear whatever I want.
5. I have the right to compassionate and informed fat-aware medical care.
6. I have the right to maintain boundaries over my body.
7. I have the right to move my body in any way I choose.
8. I have the right to live a public life without ridicule or abuse because of my body.
9. I have the right to reject diet culture.
10. I have the right to embrace the mystery of my body.

TOUCHSTONE

I HAVE THE RIGHT TO TAKE UP SPACE.

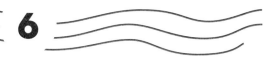

6

YOU CAN STOP SHRINKING YOURSELF

Diet culture: a cultural influence built on a fundamentally flawed way of looking at bodies, which upholds a body hierarchy based on thinness as good and fatness as bad. It is inextricably linked with other social hierarchies like race and class, and it encourages marginalization of BIPOC, the fat community, those with disabilities, those with chronic illnesses, non-male genders, those in poverty, and more.

ENCOUNTERING FREEDOM FROM DIET CULTURE is a lot like falling in love. When you meet freedom after being in a toxic relationship with diet culture for so long, it's a simultaneous breakup and a new start. It's exciting and scary and uncomfortable and delicious all at the same time. It's like meeting someone you're into at a party and them taking forever to respond to your Facebook friend request (or TikTok or whatever the kids are into these days). The joy and the impatience mingle to create an atmosphere of expectation, and at first all you can think about is the hope of truly being free. You recognize how body freedom treats you better than your ex, and slowly you see the ways that diet culture had been playing you all along, like the diets saying, "I'll be different this time" and then immediately accusing, "But if you don't lose weight, that's all on you." You'll recognize the photoshopped form-fitted figures and single chins and get angry that you ever believed a person could change their body into a work of fiction like that. Your anger is justified and will help disentangle you, even though it's exhausting and the memories of shame are painful. And there will be times when it just feels easier to go back to the way things used to be. But as your relationship with your body grows in freedom rather than restriction, you get stronger, and you get savvier at recognizing diet culture's old tricks and conceits.

We are all too familiar with the demands of diet culture. Our world has long been filled with stories of people who—according to them—have radically transformed their lives by losing weight. The average person does not question that thinness is the best and healthiest way to exist in a human body. It's what we have been trained to believe in every space, from grade school, the workplace, and the doctor's office to Hollywood, social media influencer pages, and advertisements for the diet industry.

In the natural world, diversity is a given. Trees come in sizes big and small, and flowers too. The range of differences we see in dog breeds is marvelous. However, the value that our society places on thinness has overshadowed the natural—and marvelous—phenomenon of body diversity. One of the biggest barriers to embracing nature's diversity of body size—particularly those of large size—is the medical community, which pushes the narrative that a person's weight is fully controllable through diet and exercise. It follows that if one can control one's body size, no person needs to stay fat. Thinness becomes the ideal, and thinness as a virtue has saturated every way we look at bodies, especially in medicine. But where did the cultural impulse to shrink ourselves come from?

FEARING THE BLACK BODY

Sabrina Strings traces the rise of anti-fatness in her landmark book *Fearing the Black Body: The Racial Origins of Fat Phobia*. According to Strings, our cultural obsession with thinness is rooted in white supremacy. More specifically, Strings is saying that starting in the sixteenth century, white Europeans compared themselves to the enslaved Africans they encountered. To justify their feelings of superiority, the Europeans projected that their white physiques must be superior to the African physique. That extended from a judgment on the appearance and size of their Black bodies to a judgment on the African moral character. It was projected that not only were African physical characteristics inferior in size, skin tone, and stature, but their souls were inferior too. Physical largesse became a marker for someone less cultured, less educated, and less morally upstanding.

Following this trajectory into the new world, Strings explains that as the slave trade expanded to the American colonies, white colonists continued to maintain their supposed moral superiority, expressly presented in their bodies, while at the same time denigrating Africans for their larger size. These ideas about body size and morality persist even today.

The prevailing view in the medical community is that the natural body diversity seen in fat bodies isn't natural;

it's the result of a vice. Fat people are assumed to be lazy and to lack self-control. And not just in medicine—we can clearly see how our culture at large perceives fatness by the overuse of tropes like the fat bully, the unemployed fat person, and the unattractive fat woman. A lot of people assume this reasoning against fatness is solid, based on scientific evidence showing that fatness causes poorer health outcomes. However, this assumption is wrong. In her 2011 book *Fat Shame: Stigma and the Fat Body in American Culture*, Amy Erdman Farrell traces the growth of fat phobia in media and advertising from the late nineteenth century into the twentieth. Based on her research, she writes, "What is clear from the historical documents [...] is that the connotations of the fat person—lazy, gluttonous, greedy, immoral, uncontrolled, stupid, ugly, and lacking in will power—*preceded* and then were intertwined with explicit concern about health issues."[1] The prevailing cultural dogma against fatness actually comes first; only after the bias is established does the scientific research against fatness come. These researchers make the mistake that we are emphatically warned about: correlation does not equal causation. However, they persist in assuming (or, better, demanding) that poor health outcomes are caused by fatness instead of correlated to fatness. Not only is this intellectually irresponsible and dishonest, but it is harmful on many levels.

THE PRESENT HARM OF DIET CULTURE

As we shift our attention to the present day, the work of both Strings and Farrell encourages us to be honest about what diet culture is and why it is thriving. When we talk about diet culture, we mean the cultural pressure that drives us as a society to pursue thinness at all costs. We must recognize that diet culture is built on a fundamentally flawed way of looking at bodies, one that upholds a body hierarchy that centers on thin white women and fit slender men. And it does all of this to the detriment not only of the average human being but especially to people in marginalized groups like people of color, the fat community, those with disabilities, those with chronic illnesses, those in poverty, and more.

Diet culture is racist. The sociological reason we desire thinness as a culture is specifically because we prefer white thinness over Black fleshiness. When we let the racist nature of diet culture go unchecked, it tightens the grip of racial hierarchy.

Diet culture is classist. As a seventy-billion-dollar-a-year industry, the diet business promises us results if we pay for products and gimmicks. That requires disposable income, which is unavailable to a significant portion of our society. When diet culture gets to define the terms of health, it shames those who can't afford to achieve it. This is blatantly classist. Think of the price difference between fresh fruit or vegetables and canned fruit or vegetables. Fresh produce and unprocessed foods, often touted by the diet industry as the cure-all to fatness, are largely out of reach for those in poverty. While we should be advocating for income equality and greater access to all food for those in poverty, we must also recognize that ability to participate in diet culture is reserved for those with income to spare.

Diet culture is sexist. Men and women both experience sexism within diet culture. Diet culture demands that a man be strong and muscular while also being trim and slender. It disproportionately affects women, who must strive to make themselves impossibly small, not simply physically but emotionally and intellectually too. Diet culture is part of the patriarchal apparatus that keeps women "in their place" and must be resisted. Transgender and nonbinary people also experience prejudice within diet culture. We must challenge the mindset that there is a specific way a person should look that is dependent on gender or sex. We must remember that body diversity is a natural part of human existence.

Diet culture is ableist. For people who suffer from chronic illness or disability, the promises of diet culture fall flat. One of those promises is that dieting will transform your body into one without pain or limitation. Many people are unable to eat or move in diet-guru-approved ways because of their bodies' limitations. Diet culture accuses them of not trying hard enough. When diet culture gets to define the meaning of "health and wellness," it champions strong and thin bodies and rejects weak and pained ones.

Diet culture is physically and emotionally harmful. Not only does diet culture perpetuate prejudice against people of color, those in poverty, and those in disabled and chronically ill bodies, it actively harms the people who participate in it. The research has shown repeatedly that dieting does not yield long-term success for most people.[2] In fact, dieting that causes weight fluctuation, popularly known as yo-yo dieting, increases the risk of an early death.[3] But rather than address the diet as the danger, the dieter's "lack of self-control" or "addiction to food" is blamed. That increases body shame and hatred. Also, despite abundant research on the deadliness of eating disorders, diet culture refuses to acknowledge its role in promoting disordered eating. Eating disorders are the second deadliest of mental illnesses.[4] Female adolescents who diet are eighteen times more likely to develop an eating disorder than their peers who do not diet.[5] If you need more evidence-based research on the dangers of dieting, visit the Non-Diet & Health at Every Size™ Research Library at More-Love.org.[6]

We must work to dismantle diet culture. But first we have to identify it.

IDENTIFYING DIET CULTURE

Diet culture is the sum of three parts: (1) a moral judgment of body size and shape (which, as we discussed, originated in racialized theories of body differences), (2) the belief that body size is completely controllable (through diet and exercise, and by drugs or surgery if necessary), and (3) an incentive—financial benefit, social influence, or power—to sell programs and products that promise significant body change (even though these goods and services ultimately fail to bring significant change for most people). We have the freedom to leave the diet culture practice of shrinking ourselves behind for good.

For the sake of our mental and physical health, as well as the health of those in our communities, we must cultivate the practice of asking good questions about the motivations behind the body messages we receive—financial, social, and moral motivations. We are so steeped in diet culture that at first the muck of it all can seem overwhelming, an impediment to our journey toward fat liberation. But we must remember the truth: our today body is good, even when the lies of diet culture tempt us to give up and surrender to it. Our body is good because its purpose isn't thinness or fitness or even physical health; its purpose is relationship with God, with ourselves, and with others. Leaving diet culture is the right decision, and body freedom is worth the struggle.

PACKING LIST

- ■ Questions to identify diet culture:
  - ● Does it convey the goodness of every body, or does it value thin and trim bodies over fat ones?
  - ● Does this hold all genders to the same standard?
  - ● Is this accessible to people despite their financial circumstances?
  - ● Does this make room for disabled and chronically ill bodies or uphold a skewed and ableist vision of health?
  - ● Does this recognize the roles that genetics, ability, class, and gender have in body size, or does it promise to control body size?
  - ● Who stands to benefit from this financially, socially, or morally?
  - ● Does this inspire body acceptance and freedom or body shame?

TOUCHSTONE

I CAN STOP SHRINKING MYSELF.

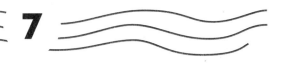

YOUR BODY IS
A STORYTELLER

Intuition: a creature's natural ability to sense its dietary,
sleep, movement, and emotional needs and to reasonably achieve them; how our body talks to us.

I WAS SITTING ON THE FLOOR of my parents' guest room
on Christmas break during grad school, dragging my fingers
across the wonderfully soft carpet. Since I wear shoes all the
time (thanks, plantar fasciitis), I didn't really get to appreciate
it much, so that day I got down next to the bed and ran my
fingers through the carpet threads. I relaxed into the floor
and studied my surroundings with a curious eye. Across
from me was a large closet, big enough to have its own set
of double doors. I noted the twin gold-colored doorknobs,
and the idea of opening doors caught my inner child's
imagination. I looked closely at the rectangular brackets at
all four corners, the hinges. And I don't know if it was me or
God or the pizza I ate the night before, but in the stillness of
my spirit, I heard these words: "Culture is the hinge that turns
the human heart from a wall into a door."

Growing up in Southern Evangelicalism, I believed that
the concept of culture was suspect. My peers and I regularly

consumed messages like "how to live for Christ in a culture of sin" and "why you should listen to Christian music instead of secular trash." Okay, they didn't say "secular trash" out loud, but it sure was implied. Back then, I'm not sure I really knew what we meant by the word "culture." I define it now as a collection of the stories we carry as a people group. And as '90s youth-group kids, our relationship with culture was binary: Christian culture was a means to evangelism and therefore good, while secular culture was the highway to hell. Our local Christian store stocked an array of T-shirts that parodied well-known icons of American culture. Well, "parodied" is too generous a word for these tees. They weren't intended to be satirical; they were meant to be cool. I had quite a few where initials were hijacked and words were replaced with propaganda, like Tommy Hilfiger morphing into "Today HeForgives" and FBI representing "Forgiven, blessed, & inspired." I was president of my high school's Christian club, Christians in Action, which of course has the initials CIA. (I used to think it was just clever and incidental that my Christian message employed the initials of an intrusive political arm of the US government, but now, relating a Christian organization for high-school students to the assassination arm of the US government is decidedly a bad choice and entirely unchristian.) For us youth-group kids of the '90s, "culture" was something inherently wrong for our in-group. We were at war with culture. We were taught to be "in, not of" culture, as if it were a byword for evil and corruption.

And yet my heart found its fingers holding tightly to the phrase "culture is the hinge." If this was true and culture was the hinge that turned the human heart into a door, "culture" couldn't simply remain a proxy for sin and licentiousness. If culture-as-hinge was true, then "culture" had depth and layers too complex—and possibly too beautiful—to write off or wage war against. That day in my parents' guest room, the realization that I had been so wrong about culture came over me like a flood. I started to see my whole life experience differently. Looking back into my own past, I could see the culture of curiosity opening my heart wall through C. S. Lewis's Pevensie children, pressing through the fur coats into the world of Narnia. I could see a culture of longing in the spoken and written confessions of love from Jane Austen's Mr. Darcy, which somehow opened Elizabeth Bennet's heart wall too. I could see how Lucy Maude Montgomery's culture of friendship cracked open my risk-averse heart for friendships of encounter like Anne's friendship with Diana Berry and Gilbert Blythe. Since that day, I've been untangling the views of my upbringing from the reality of "culture," and sometimes I feel like that word has too much baggage. And so, for our purposes, I've switched out the world "culture" for the word "story" because they really are interchangeable for me.

Richard Rohr says that the very nature of being created, of being a *thing*, is to express the spirit of the universal Christ.[1] And because the universal Christ is the original storyteller (see Hebrews 12:2), every single thing we encounter in our lives is telling us some sort of story. The soup that your mom made you when you were sick as a kid. The car that carried your firstborn home from the hospital and that got dinged on her first day with a learner's permit. It's a beautiful exercise to play with the concepts of "thing" and "story." All of the sudden, a porch light becomes a story about waiting up for your loved one returning home from a long trip. It is conversations with dear ones late into the summer evenings when even the mosquitos have gone to bed. And it's a really good marketing slogan for Motel 6.

And what would life be without story? One story is like a stone dropped in the water, the ripples moving out and out to touch all the edges of the pond. I've encountered divine swells in the stories of Rama's riding on the clouds, of Hagar's forced exile and pilgrimage, of Siddhartha's search for illumination, of Athena's gift of wisdom, and so many others in religious texts and myths. Story reaches down to our center; story draws out the beautiful knot of emotions, experiences, and efforts; story helps us untangle it all and braid it anew. Our very existence is impossible without it. The Christian tradition, too, is full of stories: The rhythm of Matthew's genealogies. Mark's focus on the grit and the glory of the march of Jesus toward Jerusalem to die. The sloppy mess of humanity of Luke's birth narrative in a barn with animals, attended by shepherds, the social pariahs of first-century Bethlehem. And from John, perhaps the most revolutionary story: that the word of God is a Person full of stories, so much more than a book or even holy scriptures. Even the story of the word we identify ourselves with— "human"—is full of life. It comes from a Proto-Indo-European root that evolves and eventually arrives in Latin as *humus*, meaning "earth" or "soil." Can you hear its story calling out to the stories inside of us? As I sit and listen for its voice, it makes me think of the words of the psalmist, deep calling out to deep. I imagine it to be quite like the sound of the kid next door calling to us, "Come outside and play—it's such a beautiful day!"

Another byproduct of growing up Southern Evangelical was that our bodies were demonized. It is commonly taught that there are three enemies of the soul: the world, the flesh, and the devil. (*The World, the Flesh, and the Devil* is also the name of a 1959 film, interestingly. That sounds either very boring or very exciting.) If within Christian teaching, "the world" is proxy for secular culture, "the flesh" is interpreted as our physical bodies, with all their wants, needs, and desires. From my post-Evangelical perspective, however, a better definition for "the flesh" is the internal impetus we all have to seek our own good above the good of others. I had hated my body for so long because I thought that hate is what God expected of me because I was "overweight" and depressed. ("Over *what* weight?" says the fat liberator in me now.) I thought that my knock knees and rough elbows were embarrassing. I thought to be a good Christian, I needed to make myself smaller—why would a godly man want to date me and eventually marry me? (That's what all my thoughts centered around at the time.) I literally prayed for a miracle where I would wake up thinner because I felt like my body was an obstacle to God's plan for my life. And I felt that way for a long time. I wouldn't be surprised to learn that *you* have also prayed for something like that. Our culture—whether it be Christian or secular or somewhere in between—demands conformity and smallness of women. That's not from God, though. God's a better storyteller than that.

MY BRADBURY YEAR

I love writing stories, especially in short story form. I wanted to work on my craft, so my husband recommended a short story collection by Ray Bradbury. I dove deep into

A Sound of Thunder and Other Stories, further solidifying my authorial crush on the guy. Then my friend Adam posted an early meme with Bradbury's face alongside this quote: "It's impossible to write 52 bad short stories in a row." In that moment, I considered myself personally challenged by Ray himself. I determined to start my Bradbury Year, a fifty-two-week-long, self-imposed writing fellowship during which I would write fifty-two short stories and travel to his hometown of Waukegan, Illinois, to let it inspire me. I aimed to eventually write a book about my experience, cleverly titled *My Bradbury Year* or *My Year with Ray,* sharing early drafts of stories, ones that sucked and ones that stunned. I already knew my thesis: story-writing is about the process, and a writer needed some transformative experience to deepen their craft. I imagined mine would be standing on the stairs of Waukegan's Carnegie Library, where the child Bradbury had read every book and gazed out at his hometown harbor on Lake Michigan. I might have made up the part about him reading every book, but . . . hagiographies, you know? It's obvious to me now that I was undertaking a pilgrimage of sorts. I just didn't realize how intensely physical a pilgrimage could be in the twenty-first century.

As I plugged along with my short story project, I started to rediscover parts of myself that had been hidden underneath the messes and distractions of motherhood. One of the reasons this could happen was bound up in the ritual of it all: Tuesday and Thursday mornings were mine. Sure, I was writing, but I was the master of my own ship with no skiffs in my wake. I convinced my best friend, Kelley, to go with me to Waukegan and do a little digging. Since I had not been in an airplane in seven years and my body had changed a lot during my three intervening pregnancies, the trip was physically a lot different than I expected. I had a middle seat on the plane, so there were two seat neighbors to think of when my fat spilled over the armrests. And that's after having hauled myself from the budget long-term parking lot through the Dallas-Fort Worth airport's miles of terminals. Still to come was getting off the plane, finding the rental car counter, and squeezing myself into the economy-sized rental car. No, I was not walking a thousand miles from France to the coast of Spain along the Way of St. James, but I was making a pilgrimage in a fat body, and I was excited and exhausted as we drove to Waukegan from O'Hare.

The local archives were not very Bradbury-heavy, surprisingly. We found his childhood home, but there was no plaque or anything to mark the genius who once lived there. We stood at the steps of the Carnegie Library and gazed out over Lake Michigan, imagining what it would have looked like through the eyes of a precocious twelve-year-old kid living through the Great Depression.

All of that took about three hours, and if I'm honest, it was a bit underwhelming. I wonder if pilgrims to holy places feel the same once they arrive and complete their rite or make their offering. However, our stomachs helped distract us from any disappointment we felt, because it was time to find a place for lunch. We ate a late lunch at a small but tantalizing Syrian place called Papa Marcos and ordered some favorites: shawarma, falafel, dolmas, tabboula salad, hummus, and baklava. Not only was the food delightful, but so was the company. The woman at the cash register, one of the owners, had her toddler with her, and Kelley and I smiled and giggled with him and missed our own kids' antics (for, like, a second—no more; we each have four kids and were glad to have a vacay).

Like any good Catholic convert, I noticed the family's Catholic art on the walls, and the woman excitedly showed me the painting of her Maronite Catholic church, located about three hours from Waukegan. She told us it was a long drive for church, but the community was full of other Syrian families, and I could tell she valued that so much. Smiling down at her son toddling around us, she said, "He is my little Sharbel, named for the saint, just like our church."

Kelley and I stayed for a little longer, enjoying our end-of-pilgrimage feast, full of food, chatting like best friends do. That's probably a common experience of pilgrims, resting and refueling, body and soul, after a long journey. When the time came to leave, we bid Sharbel and his mom farewell, and we hopped in our rental car to drive down that same shoreline into Chicago, where my sister lived. We had a blast with my sister and her husband, doing touristy things, including celebrating my thirty-second birthday with dessert on one of the top floors of the Hancock Building (though it's called something else now). The trip was a smashing success, but I admit that my pilgrimage to Bradbury's hometown felt silly, even foolish, as a thing in itself. I couldn't see yet that my love for Ray was just a spark for this pilgrimage that awaited me, body and soul. For my body, the travel limitations I experienced during my Bradbury Year pressed me to fight for accessibility in travel and accommodation. In my soul, well . . . for now, suffice it to say that physical and mental anguish can make you question if your life even matters at all. Many years later, I can see how my soul began to grow into its fuller self—my fuller self—on that trip.

My body's goodness and its pain mingle together in nearly every moment, thanks to chronic pain and post-COVID-19 syndrome. Acknowledging that my body is a trustworthy storyteller helps me resist the lie that the presence of pain makes the goodness invalid. In our bodies—today, just as they are—we carry our story with us, and in a very real way, our bodies tell our stories. Our bodies are trustworthy storytellers, which is especially important when diet culture feeds us manipulated narratives and false promises of thin happiness. My body tells a story of joy, sadness, life, grief, delight, trauma, pleasure, and love. And so does yours.

PACKING LIST

- ■ My body is a storyteller: I need the right questions about the story my body is telling.
  - ● What story is my body telling?
  - ● How does that story differ from the one I believe about my body?
  - ● How can I listen more to my body's good story, even if pain comes along with that story?
  - ● Does the idea of pilgrimage help you see your body's story more clearly?

■ Sit or stand in front of a mirror. Look at yourself with tender eyes. What story do you see? Is that a true story? If not, what is the true story? What lies have you been believing about the story your body is telling?

─────── **TOUCHSTONE** ───────

MY BODY IS A TRUSTWORTHY STORYTELLER.

8

CURIOSITY IS YOUR BODY'S FRIEND

Body shame: the invisible burden of embarrassment, grief, and disappointment caused by a misplaced concern that your body doesn't measure up to someone's ideal body standards.

THE NOTICING™ (NOT REALLY TRADEMARKED ... I'M JUST BEING DRAMATIC)

The human body is worthy of our trust. That's a hell of a statement, but I've come by it honestly. I can trust my body. The shadows in my life convinced me that trusting my body was the very thing I *couldn't* do. I made external rules that paid little attention to how they made my body feel. Even worse, there were times when I treasured the feeling of hunger pangs because I believed I was punishing my body, disciplining it into submission and smallness. Finding my way out of the shadows began with something very simple: noticing. And I noticed that whenever I tried to make myself smaller, my will never cooperated for long. I thought the answer was to pray for more will power. But that didn't seem to help either.

When I was pregnant with my fourth baby, my OBGYN told me that bread was the culprit for my body's size. But whenever I avoided bread, it called my mental phone number more often than the extended-car-warranty people: "We are calling to inform you that your carbohydrate count is about to be depleted. If you want to be connected to Bread, please press one." With every ring, my anti-bread resolve weakened, and by the seventy-sixth attempt, I could not keep myself from pressing one a bajillion times in a row.

One fateful day, hunger led me to the fridge to find a bread alternative. Of course, all I could think about was bread. Normally, I would push that desire down into the pit of my stomach, but today was different. Instead of shunning my desire for bread, I held it in my mind's eye and looked at it, truly noticed it. All of a sudden, The Noticing showed me that whenever I restrict bread, all I can think about is eating bread. Maybe it wasn't just me sucking at self-control. Maybe that was just how my brain worked. So if restricting bread makes me want more bread, why wouldn't I just stop restricting? Ah, yes—the body size thing. But attempting to make myself smaller by restricting wasn't working.

Seriously, consider the history of bread. (In my deepest theatrical voice☺ Since the dawn of civilization . . . oh, wait. I'm not a freshman in College Comp 101. In my regular speaking voice:) Until recently, about halfway through the twentieth century, the concept of bread has signified abundance, access, and affordability. Consider the importance of bread in Egyptian culture. Ancient Egyptians were buried with loaves of it to sustain them on the journey to the afterlife. Modern Egyptians use the same word, *aish*, for bread and for life. (Personal LOL: Jesus saying, "I am the bread of breads." Talk about being the BOAT, the breadest of all time.) I know it's considered gauche to quote an online dictionary in a serious piece of writing (I'm not in freshman comp anymore), but this explanation of bread's symbolism from Encyclopedia.com is so 🔥 that I have to share it:

> Whether it is leavened or unleavened, made into loaves or cakes, baked, steamed, or fried in oil, bread is universal. Whatever the grain, bread occupies an important place in every civilization. It has exceptional nutritional value, and as the only near perfect product for human nourishment, can be consumed by itself.[1]

Wow. Allow me to gather my thoughts as I slow clap whoever wrote that prose. Bread *is* universal! Bread *is* nearly perfect! Why have we let anti-fat bias and diet culture corrupt this view of bread? It deserves a place of honor in our cultural imagination, not demonization. Bread is life. And I was being asked to give up life so that I could (maybe) make myself smaller. Before The Noticing, I hadn't been able to see that restriction, specifically of bread, is what sent me to the abyss. I was forcing my body into a bread famine. Bread—the thing Jesus describes himself as in the Gospels— is a good thing. If it's a staple, it's probably not a good idea to cut it out of your food choices (unless you have a medical issue that requires you to do so).

Thankfully, The Noticing showed me the connection between restriction of a specific food and a shame spiral that sent me to rock bottom. Logically speaking, if I hated shame cycling about my body because of the food I do or don't eat, I had to stop engaging in the shame spiral's cause—restriction. I know that's a revolutionary idea in this culture that attempts to control bodies, especially female bodies, by demanding that we take up less space. But I could see, more clearly than ever, that attempts to do this were literally harmful. So I did it: I gave up restricting, and in doing so, slowly but surely, I have found a measure of freedom I never dreamed was possible. I ditched restriction and forced exercise and body shame because I intuitively realized how damaging they were for me. I guess I joined the fat liberation movement before I had even heard of it.

MY EXPERIENCE OF THE SHAME CYCLE

Before The Noticing, bread restriction propelled me into a scarcity mentality, where I ate every single grain of wheat I could find. It was like my body intuited that a bread shortage was coming and knew it needed to stock up. That mentality prompted me to eat far past fullness, which led to physical discomfort, which dragged me into blame and anger at myself. Down I went, around and around, stuck in a whirlpool that sucked me into the abyss. The abyss had a name: Rejection and Unworthiness. When I arrived there, I truly believed that I was fundamentally unworthy of being loved and that I would always been worthy of rejection because of my body. I want to share how I learned to climb out of the abyss, but first let's identify some landmarks on the downward spiral.

1. **Triggering event**
   Something in my life causes me to panic, whether I know it or not. Sometimes it's obvious; sometimes it's subtle. Food restriction is one of the primary ways I slide into the spiral. Even the idea or suggestion of restriction can send me spinning. Because I have such a history with restriction, my body immediately tries to save me, and I feel a biological need to stock up on whatever I might consider

restricting. Another trigger for me is feeling pain in any part of my body, but especially if the pain could possibly be related to body shape or size. Your trigger could be a negative comment about your body, clothes not fitting, or something seemingly unconnected to food and body issues. Every trigger is legitimate and worth investigating.

The Shame Spiral

1. Triggering Event	2. Response
Restriction of chips and salsa	Eat all the chips and salsa!

2. **Response**
   In an effort to protect my body, my psyche recognizes that I am entering into a phase where something vital will be restricted, whether it be bread, chips and salsa, or cake. Whenever I encounter this food—in the flesh or in my brain—my psyche drives me to eat as much of it as I can because it doesn't know when this important life source will be available to me again. It's a protective measure, but it can literally feel like I am not in control of myself. To a certain extent, I'm not—my psyche is.

3. **Observation**
   I notice which feelings—physical or emotional—my response causes in me. If I have eaten past the point of fullness, I can experience physical pain in my abdomen that makes sitting or lying down extremely challenging. This can also include acid reflux. Emotionally, eating chips and salsa past fullness also makes me feel anger toward

myself for a perceived lack of self-control.

The Shame Spiral

3. Observation	4. Wishful Thinking
I am in pain or major discomfort.	If only I had more self-control.

4. **Wishful thinking**

   I think everyone has a picture in their mind's eye of what a perfect life would be, right? And if circumstances were just the way I wanted, I would have no problems at all. My imaginary perfect life often involves a specific form of self-control and the ability to perfectly regulate my intake and output. I admit that I have believed that intake/output self-control could lead me to a state of happiness where my energy level, BMI, clothing size, body shape, and sex drive are perfect. This is certainly a hypothesis that many people in our society have faith in. But what happens when this hypothesis is proven false after being tested over and over and over again, failing more than 90 percent of the time? If I continue to believe in the hypothesis, I am guilty of wishful thinking—or believing in a reality that is contradicted by the facts. It is wishful thinking to believe that all my problems would be solved if I had more self-control.

5. **Assigning Blame**

   Oof. When I am in pain, the burden of blame nearly suffocates me. If I believe I am responsible for the pain I am enduring, then I could have done something to prevent it. But I didn't, and that's on me. This kind of blame makes asking for help nearly impossible. An inner voice of anger charges me with irresponsibility, or even apathy, toward my body. And that voice is confirmed by all the trolls (and sometimes people I'm close to) telling me that if I cared about my body, I should do something about it. The suggestions they offer look bleak to me: a starvation diet, good food/bad food restriction lists, punishing exercise, and even stomach amputation. Diet culture tries to downplay its severity by calling it other names, but it still fundamentally alters a healthy, functioning, and necessary organ. After the majority of your stomach is amputated, the remaining stomach tissue is sewn together like a sleeve, a tube connecting your esophagus to your pyloric sphincter. That is mutilation. That is an act of violence toward a human body. And it is offered to fat patients like (sugar-free) candy in a sweets shop.

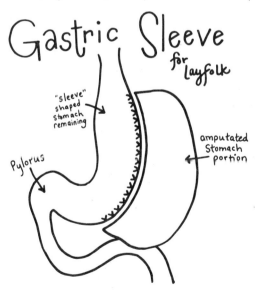

If you have had this surgery, I hope you can hear that I am not judging you for choosing it; we are all masters of our own bodies and are free to do what we want. What I take issue with is that this extremely serious procedure is pushed on fat patients (and some not-so-fat ones) while (1) someone is making lots of money on it, and (2) there is so little evidence that it "works" long term (i.e., helps people become and stay smaller for the rest of their lives). Also, we have been taught through the media and in our relationships that fat people are fat because of laziness, stupidity, and lack of discipline. And it is when I internalize those thoughts about myself that I begin to believe that my pain is my fault. As a fat person, I am specifically susceptible to the belief that my body size indicates my moral character. I counter this lie with the truth: body size is morally neutral, and I am not in pain because I deserve it. If I am unable to recognize this, I am further trapped by shame.

The Shame Spiral

5. Assigning Blame	6. Negative Projection
This pain is all my fault.	Pain and discomfort are my destiny.

6. **Negative projection**
   At this point in the spiral, I tend to make a judgment about my future, based on how I feel and who I believe is responsible for all of it. In this place, I am prone to

believe that "this too shall pass" does not apply to me. My therapist and I have been working on these negative projections for a while. (Thanks, Stacey! You're awesome.) When I get into that pool of negativity, I can't climb out until I grab on to an anchor. Sometimes it takes the form of a mantra like this: "Just because it sucks right now doesn't mean it will suck forever."

7. **The pit of despair**
   If hope eludes me, despair overwhelms me, and I enter the pit of despair. I feel it at my very core: I am nothing. I am not worthy of love or time or attention. I will never find acceptance. This abyss causes a numbness that prevents me from believing anything different. I have been here often, as a fat person, as a creative person, as a writer. I'm also married to an academic, so we have almost suffocated in the ether of existential nothingness while we ponder the concepts of vocation and nihilism. (Who, me? I'm not dramatic. Not at all.) The only way out of the abyss that I have found is to ground myself. A therapist friend taught me one way to do this—as I sit in the abyss, first I find five things I can literally see. Now four things I can hear. Three things I can touch. Two things I can smell. One thing I can taste. This practice draws me back to my physical body after I have alienated her out of shame. Another is this: I inhale deeply through my nose and then let my breath out slowly and say, "This is my body." I can say it several times, with each repetition emphasizing a different word. "This is *my* body. *This* is my body. This is my *body*. This *is* my body." Shame alienates us from our bodies on

our way into the abyss, so it follows that an intentional reunion of body and soul provides purchase for our feet as we climb out of it.

The Shame Spiral

7. The Pit of Despair

I believe that I am responsible for my pain, but I don't know how to address it. I wallow in the despair that I have no hope for comfort or joy in my life.

TURNING POINTS

Feelings and observations of feelings can be neutral. An observation about your body or your appetite can be very powerful, for good or for ill. Learning to observe my body in a neutral and curious way is super important when I find myself slipping into shame. If I hit the observation level of the shame spiral described above and can choose curiosity instead of judgment, the results are astounding. Experiencing difficulties within our bodies, whether they are physical (like joint aches or tight clothing) or emotional (rejection and disappointment), we are culturally conditioned to embrace shame and blame for whatever it is. But what if I could observe that pain or discomfort and respond to it with curiosity instead of shame? If I think, "Jeez, my midsection hurts," I could condemn my body and start the shame spiral. Or I can hold that thought in my mind and look at it with curiosity:

- *Why* am I hurting?
  - Is my clothing restricting blood flow?

- Did I not notice getting a bruise somewhere?
- Am I getting sick?
- Could this be connected to a medicine I am taking?
- Could this be connected to a physical change I've recently undergone?

■ *How* could I stop hurting?

- Invest in looser clothing?
- Change my sitting position?
- Do I need to be treated for an illness?
- Try a different treatment?
- Try a difference physical activity?

All of these questions can be asked from a neutral, inquisitive position rather than a judgmental, shame-inducing one. If I am able to recognize pain and question it, I might be able to avoid the shame spiral completely. However, sometimes I don't realize that I'm in the spiral until I'm several revolutions in. Even then, not all is lost—I can identify where I am in the spiral and put on the brakes with the responses shown in the illustration above. I also pair all of this with regular therapy and honest talks with good friends.

Wishful thinking antidote: When I arrive at the wishful thinking part of the spiral, I can find ways to turn from shame to curiosity too. There is so much about weight science that we do not know. Body size and shape are influenced by genetics, class, racist structures, and more. Just taking one of those aspects, genetics, helps me break down my tendency toward wishful thinking. I can't force my way out of my genetics, right? And even if I could, how can I be sure that whatever problems I have are actually caused by a lack of self-control? Finding my way out of harmful wishful thinking begins by asking: What problems do I think this will solve? Once I have a list of problems I believe can be solved by my wishful thinking, I must follow up by asking: Will this actually solve these specific problems? Usually not. But once I can see that wishful thinking won't solve my problems, I can get to investigating true, reliable solutions that will actually make my life better. Remember, curiosity is our friend.

The way out of blame: The way out of bearing the blame for your body's pain deals with the universal nature of pain, and, again, curiosity is our friend. I ask myself, "Do people in thin bodies have pain like this?" The answer is always yes. As far as I have seen, there is no physical pain unique to fatness. Every human on earth experiences pain. I also must remember that medical and cultural fat phobia perpetuates the lie that pain is solely the individual's responsibility. The truth is that systemic, institutionalized anti-fat bias contributes to fat people's pain when a majority of health-care providers believe this lie of individual responsibility for pain too. We push back against this systemic injustice by demanding evidence-based health care that sees fatness as morally neutral.

Glimmer of hope: If I don't have a "right now is not forever" truth to fall back on when pain and circumstances stink up my life, I flounder and sink into despair. I am weighed down by sorrow and self-pity. My bones literally ache, and my stomach sours with existential angst to which I can see no end. The only thing that can pull me from this desolate place is to try to find some glimmer of hope. The only way out of the abyss that I have found is to ground myself, using the breathing techniques I described above. If you've never arrived at this glimmer of hope, I trust that the truths in this book will give you your first glimpse.

CHILDLIKE CURIOSITY

Kids are amazing when it comes to curiosity and bodies. "Mommy, why are you fat?" is a question I have encountered from at least three of my four kiddos. Once I have made the shift my own heart and mind about my body and curiosity, I can hear that question with the curiosity it contains. Instead of shushing them when they ask a genuine question—giving them the idea that talking about bodies is wrong, especially fat ones—it lets them explore body concepts and embrace their bodies' goodness from the beginning. If you're worried that you have already introduced barriers to their curiosity, don't fret. We can start this journey anywhere, and so can they.

These are some examples of scenarios I have experienced with my own kids where I have tried to encourage curiosity instead of judgment:

A child notices that someone is fat. What does that word mean to you, buddy? Where have you heard that word before? Is it okay to be fat? Well, you know what we say—all bodies are good bodies!

A child says someone has called them fat. How did that make you feel? Did the person who said it mean to give you a compliment, or were they trying to make you feel bad about your body? You know what? Fat bodies are good bodies!

A child sees or hears a negative fat trope in the media.
I noticed that this character made the other character feel
bad about the size of their body. Do you think that was okay?
What would you tell that character if you could?

Learning to trust our bodies is an invitation as much as
it is a challenge. Can you imagine how your life could have
been different if intuition wasn't trained out of you? If
using curiosity to stop the shame spiral had been modeled
for you? I have good news: using the tools of curiosity
and climbing out of the shame cycle, we can model
that trust for our own inner child and find freedom from
shame.

PACKING LIST

- How to climb out of the body-shame spiral.
  Learn to identify the landmarks of the spiral:
  1. Triggering Event
  2. Response
  3. Observation
  4. Wishful Thinking
  5. Assigning Blame
  6. Negative Projection
  7. The Pit of Despair
     - Insert curiosity at whatever level you find
       yourself at. Ask good questions of your
       responses and emotions. Over time, you will
       learn to recognize the shame spiral close to its
       start, and often you can more easily prevent
       yourself from slipping down the path, climbing
       out from wherever you find yourself in it.

■ Questions and statements to use when the conversation turns to fatness, whether that happens at home or in public:

1. Make no assumptions.
   - The first time my daughter called me fat, she had no idea that the term could be offensive. When children ask loud questions or make comments about bodies, make sure you understand their mindset before offering a corrective. Kids aren't fat phobic until they are taught to be.

2. Approach with curiosity.
   - I try to respond with a question that needs more than a yes/no answer, such as "Oh, yeah? What does that mean to you?" I let the child explain what the word "fat" means to them, and then I go from there with a question like "Do you think it's okay to be fat? Why or why not?"

3. Examine personal biases.
   - The children around me will pick up on the way I view my body and other bodies. I must continue to work on my own bias against fatness so that it does not transfer to them.

4. Reinforce truth.
   - The barrage of diet-culture negativity will threaten to overwhelm any fat-positive foundation I am laying with the kids in my life, so I almost always end conversations about bodies with this call and response:

Me: And what do we say about bodies? (wait)
Me and child: All bodies are good bodies!

- Your own call and response could be any variation of this truth. Come up with it in your community, whether that's in your family, in your classroom, or in children's church.

TOUCHSTONE

CURIOSITY IS MY BODY'S FRIEND.

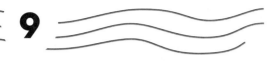

9

YOUR BODY IS YOUR HOME

Fat hospitality: the act of creating welcome private and public spaces for fat bodies, including adequate seating, access to facilities, and an atmosphere of fat acceptance.

IN THE CHAPTER ABOUT OUR BODIES as trustworthy storytellers, we spoke about changing our view of our bodies from roadblock to door and that stories add hinges to any wall to turn it into a door. Perhaps the door was locked before, but now we can push with our curious fingertips and find that it gives way before us. But what is it a door to? If I stand and look at the door on its hinges, craning my neck to see around it, I realize it's a house. And my body's not just the door; it is the whole structure. It's got a wraparound porch with great big rocking chairs inviting me to sit. Green plants hang from the porch rafters, and lights glow from within, shining out of the hand-hammered glass windows. It's full of life. It's full of . . . me.

The door opens to my touch. I walk in and feel like it is home, though one I've not fully inhabited in a long time. My current favorite color—lilac purple—adorns the entryway walls, and I stand in the anteroom with a sense of anticipation, excitement I've not often known. Suddenly, though, I stop—my feet won't move down the hallway because, well, this is me, and I know that there could be parts I'm not ready to confront. But something about the sound of the music coming from the living room and the smell of bread emanating from the kitchen promises beauty amid whatever lies ahead. I wander into the kitchen, cut off a slice of fresh-baked bread, and slather it with butter. I pour myself a cup of tea and take my snack across the hall to the living room. I make myself comfortable in a big armchair, delighted in myself as the sounds of Ella Fitzgerald and Billie Holiday float from the record player in the background.

"Comfortable"—it comes from the Latin *com*, which means "with," and *fort*, which means "strength." Being at home with myself, with this body of mine, truly does give me strength. I am offering fat hospitality to myself. In this home of my body, it's okay to be fat. I breathe a deep sigh of relief, air that filled my lungs and expanded my fat belly now released slowly as I sit with eyes closed. Home.

Your body is not a fixer-upper. Have you ever been house shopping and seen one that made you think, "That house needs a lot of work to make it beautiful," and all of a sudden your mind is filled with images of wrecking balls and bulldozers? Then there are houses that catch your eye, and even if they need work, you know you don't have to make it beautiful—you just need to draw the beauty out. If bodies are like houses, your body isn't the former, the fixer-upper purchased at a reduced price. No, finding a home within yourself is like investing in the beauty of a house that doesn't need demolition, but rather, care. Your body-home isn't in a race with the Joneses down the street for the best home competition. That league play is all disappointing fantasy anyway.

A note about Christian diet culture: the way that Christians have spoken of bodies in the past hundred years is fundamentally flawed, their "your body is a temple" nonsense, taken out of context and used to manipulate people into sculpting and toning instead of loving and abiding. As a Christian, I do believe that God delights in making a home *with* me and *within* me. How that happens is a mystery, but what God doesn't do is come in and make a mental list of what I need to fix. I think that what God notices about our body-home is the bones of the house, the attention to detail its designer paid it, and the promise of abundant life that echoes through its halls. I've come to know God as one who urges us toward self-giving love for our neighbors and ourselves as we do justly, love mercy, and walk humbly with God (see Micah 6:8). I see nowhere in Scripture where God asks us to make ourselves physical specimens to serve our neighbors—quite the opposite. God uses the weakness of the world, the bodies that others reject, as the instruments of divine love. So as we come to find a home within our own bodies, let's toss out the "diet devotionals," as J. Nicole Morgan calls them—the books that tell you how to use religion to shrink yourself, with titles like *Weight Loss, God's Way* and *Faithfully Fit*. Let's replace them with thick, rich, indulgent books bound in beautiful fabrics, little pieces of abundance making up a part of our abundant home.

SHADOW ON A TIGHTROPE AND THE '80s

At the beginning of the 1980s, the fat liberation movement continued to take root, even though it had a hard time finding its home. On the East Coast, Freespirit (also known as Vivian Mayer) worked with Judith Stein and Diane Denne to organize the first Feminist Fat Activist Working Meeting, which took place in April of 1980. That conference marked a transition in the movement. Freespirit turned her focus to graduate school, and the work and legacy of Fat Liberator Publishing landed in the lap of Lisa Schoenfielder. Lisa, a fat woman, partnered with Barb Wieser, a thin woman, to edit an anthology titled *Shadows on a Tightrope: Writings by Women on Fat Oppression*. As the foundation for the anthology, they used both published writings and previously unpublished pieces from Fat Liberator Press. In 1983, *Shadow on a Tightrope* debuted with a foreword by Judy Freespirit, in which she preserved a large part of the history of the fat liberation movement that you read in this book today. In the book, fat women shared their perspectives on fat myths, fat legacies, and social stigma that excluded fat people from activities like dancing and sports, enduring harassment and isolation, medical violence toward fat folk, and seeing fat women as survivors of all of this. To me, this book is precious—and I mean that in a "precious jewel" way, not a "precious moments" way—because it tells me so much of my story, even though it came out the year before my birth. In recent history, fat women have always needed to be survivors. It's a part of who we are.

For the remainder of the '80s, fat liberation continued in scattered places around the United States. Across the Atlantic, though, things were happening as well. In Great Britain, the London Fat Women's Group began to discuss fat liberation in the British feminist press. The 1989 conference organized by the group was widely covered (pun always intended) by

British media. Fat Women's Group cofounder Heather Smith describes the experience: "For a few hours we stepped out of our isolation and into an unfamiliar reality. It felt like the alchemy of other fat women's energy collected and combined and strengthened us all in ways we are not used to. The world was different; it was exciting and emotional and scary. I know the way I felt for days afterwards was different from anything before or since: a brief glimpse of what it might feel like not to be oppressed."[1] These fat women found a home in community with each other, which allowed them to feel more at home in their bodies. But the world around them couldn't offer the same hospitality, so the group dissipated.

All of this, along with an episode of the BBC program *Open Space* called "Fat Women Are Here to Stay," caught the eye of Charlotte Cooper, who would go on to become a giant in fat activism (yes, I know). But in the aftermath of the London Fat Women's Group conference, there was no group for Cooper to join, and so she tried to restart what had previously existed. Aside from a popular newsletter, due to her inexperience and group dynamics, the group didn't last longer than a few years.[2] As most of British fat activism in the early '90s moved in a more body-positive direction (using today's understanding of the term), it was less about the issues of fat political issues like discrimination and lack of access, and more about making oneself feel good about one's body.[3] In itself, that is not a bad thing—it's wonderful to have good feelings for your body, and finding a home in your body gradually enables more positive feelings, which helps spur more liberation. But if a movement is not at least in part about accessibility, valuable people get left behind no matter how they feel. We need both for fat liberation to be achievable and sustainable.

WELCOME TO THE NEIGHBORHOOD

Having found myself at home with myself—even with the dark and painful parts of me—I began to notice the neighboring houses. I remember reading an article in *Christianity Today* called "God Loves My Fat Body as It Is," by J. Nicole Morgan. Her words about being fat and still loved by God resonated so deeply within me that I knew I needed more of what she had to say. From our first conversation, it felt like Nicole was living in the same neighborhood as me—right next door, even. She was several years ahead of me on her fat liberation journey, and she helped me articulate my purpose on the journey—to find peace with my body and to help others do the same. It was Nicole who introduced me to the term "fat acceptance." I had no idea that other fat people were and had been extensively dialoguing about fat dignity, literally for decades.

Nicole modeled what it meant to be a fat advocate in a thin-obsessed world, and she taught me what HAES stood for (health at every size). She pointed me to look inward to confront my ableist thoughts, that health could ever be considered the highest aim of my humanity. She shaped my life as I now live it. If this sounds like a hagiography of J. Nicole Morgan to you, you're not far off. Nicole is as close to a fat liberation saint as there has ever been seen. Her self-described leadership style of "I'll go first" opened up space for me to fumble through my own first attempts at fat liberation and activism.

It was an honor to cohost the *Fat & Faithful* podcast with her as we both wrote and spoke about our journeys to accept our bodies, specifically as Christians in the fat acceptance world. Her book *Fat and Faithful: Learning to Love Our Bodies, Our Neighbors, and Ourselves* is a must-read. If you've heard me speak about gluttony before, I got that definition from Nicole. If God frames God's whole world around self-giving neighbor love, we must build our own theology from a bedrock of neighbor love. Nicole, working from this frame of mind, reworked the definition of gluttony from its commonplace understanding of "eating too much" or, more generically, "overconsumption."

If we merely define gluttony as consuming "too much," we must ask ourselves, who is to say what is *too much*? The scientists who determine serving size? Or the CEOs of weight-loss companies? There are far too many variables here—cultural practices, outdated or misinterpreted science and data, and so much more. But the foundational measure for people of the Christian faith is neighbor care. In her definition of gluttony, Nicole Morgan partnered this neighbor-oriented understanding with the liberation message that frees the marginalized: gluttony is consumption that harms our neighbor. Two slices of cake or more at a birthday party? Not oppressing anyone, unless you took someone else's slice, leaving them none. Demanding that underpaid fast-food workers return to work without paying them more and while denying them health-care coverage during a pandemic? That is consumption that harms our neighbor. That is gluttony. I do want to note, as Morgan often does, that there is no ethical consumption under capitalism; unregulated supply chains inevitably deny just wages and enforce cruel working conditions at some point along the way. (Just research "fast-food chain tomatoes" to learn about injustice against tomato farmers.[4])

My point is that what we have been taught about gluttony is all wrong. In fact, feasting is an important part of our lives—both spiritual and communal. When we gather to celebrate, to mourn, to welcome, or to send off, we are living out our calling as people of God. And there's not a calorie limit on this calling. I hope to God that the Divine is not that petty. No, people of the Christian faith aren't called to live by food laws that account for every jot and tiddle. We are called to freedom, as a people—as a community. Liberation is the way of Jesus—loving and freeing our neighbors as we love and free ourselves from oppression and harmful consumption. These things are not based on an American sense of rough individualism; no, they are deeply rooted in community. We are not alone. You are not alone. I love how Jesus tells us he is making a home for us and that it's gonna be a block party with many homes (John 14: 2–3). What if the home Jesus is preparing is us, in our bodies? We are being invited to settle in more deeply and profoundly than we ever could have imagined, in our own bodies.

Meeting Nicole was a watershed moment in my life. She helped me shift my fat-aware focus from just myself to a self-and-neighbor framework for fat activism. It wasn't just her redefinition of gluttony that caused this moment in my life. It was her connection to the fat community. Solidarity is the bond between people who have shared life experiences, and there isn't anything like it in the world. Sure, I can talk about my fat troubles with my smaller-bodied friends, and I can know that they care for me and sympathize, but when I am speaking with another fat person, we connect on a different level. Such solidarity is what the fat community offers to us—people in bodies like ours, who experience the same prejudice and exclusion, and who have survived. Within the fat community, there is a sea of vast resources that enrich and support the life of the fat person. Once we can embrace our bodies as our home, we can explore the neighborhood and live a richer and fuller life, together.

PACKING LIST

- Use your imagination to enter the door of your body and look around. What parts of you do you need to embrace? What rooms surprise you? What rooms do you want to feel more at home in?
- Once you're at home in your body, check out the neighborhood! Finding fat community is vital, particularly when it comes to specialized communities on social media such as:
  - Fat fashion
  - Fat sex
  - Fat romance
  - Fat accessibility
  - Fat-aware medical care
  - General fat community
  - My Facebook group, All Bodies Are Good Bodies, is a good place to start!

--- TOUCHSTONE ---

MY BODY IS MY HOME.

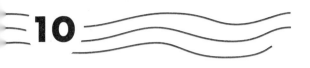

YOUR BODY IS BEAUTIFUL AND COMPLEX

> **Binary: related to or composed of two things, like the common Christian understanding of the human person as body and soul or flesh and spirit.**

WHEN I DISCOVERED THAT I WASN'T ALONE, that fat people all over had the same drive for body justice that I did, my world changed. It was almost like the plot of Amy Poehler's 2021 film *Moxie*, where the teenage Vivian discovers her mother's former life of feminist activism during the '90s—in particular when Vivian discovers the *zine*, a newsletter-like publication handed out at feminist punk-rock concerts in the early '90s. I discovered that fat liberation had its own zine scene, started by fat activist and mother of the modern fat liberation movement, Marilyn Wann. Her zine *Fat?So!*, advertised by mail order in feminist magazines, amassed a huge following and empowered countless fat women to embrace their fat identities. As *Fat?So!* readership grew in its photocopied glory (literally, it was just photocopied in black and white), the rise of the internet in the late '90s and early 2000s also opened the way for fat bloggers like Marianne Kirby, with her blog *The Rotund*, to accrue fat followers interested in fat identity and fashion. Challenging society's conventional wisdom that thinness was superior to fatness, the authors of these zines and blogs celebrated fatness and resisted the traditional competition among women, thinness versus fatness. They celebrated fatness. Reading the writing of these women nearly thirty years later was a revelation.

BUSTING BINARIES

You've heard it said that nature abhors a vacuum? Well, I say that humans abhor a spectrum . . . but we love binaries. White and black, old and young, clean and dirty. In fact, we base so much of our lives on binaries that we employ them as rudimentary building blocks to construct our world for children. Binaries can be helpful in many applications; hot and cold, for example, are very important to learn, especially when it comes to avoiding cooking surfaces. Yes and no, good and bad, something and nothing. We crave a binary. It helps us keep track of things. Our brains crave the structure that binaries offer.

For much of my life, I assumed this was how morality worked: to know what to do, I needed to know what not to do. How could I live a good life if I didn't learn how to avoid living a bad one? And the thing about binaries is that they are very hard to take apart. I see them like the lines in a grid I make in my head to give me clues and expectations about the world when I am in new situations. Everything has to line up. I remember being in a Barnes & Noble bookstore several years ago, inspecting the cover of a book about maps. I opened the book and flipped to a page where the author asked a question: What direction is South America in relation to North America? Well, I was confident that I knew! South America was due south of North America. A simple page turn revealed the right answer in map form, and it proved the map in my head wrong. Despite what my binary-loving brain told me about the location of North America and South America, the latter is actually significantly southeast from the former. If you go due south from almost any part of the United States, you end up in the depths of the Pacific Ocean, not in Brazil or Argentina like my brain-projected map told me. North and south. My brain, categorizing machine that it is, took two geographical locations diagonally situated to each other and overrode what was actual reality. The words trumped the actual physical relationship, I believe, because the brain prefers neat and tidy organization to messy, diagonal, interconnected reality. Binaries make that way easier.

It's remarkable how unsettled we get when we are presented with information that disrupts our dearly held binaries. Think about the recognized sexes in our species. From time immemorial, we have separated the human species into two groups: has penis and has no penis. Those who can bear and nurse children, and those who can neither bear children nor nurse them. However, the field of genetics shows us that we need more than a binary. We need at least three categories when talking about biological sex: male, female, and varieties of intersex individuals who don't fit into the male or female column. And the biological categories don't begin to capture the incredible diversity of human gender expression. But even when the scientific evidence is clear, as a society we are quick to commit violence—physical, mental, emotional, spiritual—on humans who biologically do not fit the binary. (Again, to make this clear, I'll repeat that intersex humans have not changed their biological sex; it's simply how their genes came out from the genetic swimming pool that is started in the procreative act.) But our first response is fear, which quickly grows into violence and ostracization of the "misfit." We love our binaries, and we enforce them with whatever it takes. But there is a more excellent way.

FLESH BAD, SPIRIT GOOD?

I grew up as a Protestant Christian, attending a Bible church all through childhood and then a spirit-filled, missionary-making, nondenominational church in college. I learned a lot of beautiful things along the way, a love for the Christian scriptures and the charismatic ecstasies of praise and worship chief among them. But I also imbibed the idea that my body, the flesh, is bad and must be tamed by the spirit. My pastor in college literally called his body "this old fleshcan." I already felt uncomfortable and alienated from my body (because I am a human living in the twenty-first century). His words just gave me more of a reason to see my body as a disgusting metal receptacle seeping trash juice, in which I waited and begged for Jesus to come rescue me.

It's no surprise that the "smells and bells" of the Catholic Church spoke volumes to my body; my nose, ears, eyes, skin, and tongue could receive the Good News with joy just as much as my heart and mind and soul. It was in becoming

Catholic that I could heartily say that my body's not a trashy soul container—my body is me, and without its beauty, I would not be able to know God. (I'm definitely not saying one must become Catholic to embrace the truth; it's just how it worked out for me.) I wrote about all that jazz more in depth in my first book, *Lovely: How I Learned to Embrace the Body God Gave Me* (Our Sunday Visitor, 2018).

JESUS, THE BINARY-BUSTER

Consider the beauty of the rainbow or the glimmer of light filtering through a prism. If the light spectrum were flattened into just two options, blinding white or pitch black, the loss would be devastating. We tend to think that an A-or-B, us-or-them framework simplifies and protects. But in flattening the realities of human experience into binaries, we actually lose more than we gain. We're afraid to let go of a life of either/or, and that fear often expresses itself in violence: the Catholic and Protestant divide in Ireland, the anti-Semitic crusade to perfect the Aryan race in Nazi Germany, the genocide of the Tutsis by the Hutus in Rwanda, the violence by straight people against the LGBTQIA community, the brutalization of Black Americans by white supremacists in the United States. If a person or a group of people—even by simply existing— are subject to the viciousness of the "order" imposed and supported by binaries, how much worse the implications for those who actively resist and defy them.

"The incarnation of Jesus rejects the binary." When my friend and body liberation advocate Patrilie Hernandez said this to me, it resounded in my core. It had come up in a conversation between Patrilie and her partner, who, like me, is Catholic. In Catholicism, we repeat over and over again that Jesus is God and human at the same time, forever. We believe that by becoming a human being—born miraculously to an unwed teenager and enfleshing Christ (the second person of the mysterious Trinity), Jesus resists the gnostic dualism of a flesh-bad, spirit-good binary. (Which, by the way, was condemned by early Christians as heresy.) We Catholics literally celebrate this binary-busting every time a Mass is offered. We eat and drink the body and blood of Jesus, truly present in the bread and wine. We put a physical piece of Jesus in our mouths, chewing and swallowing. Our saliva—one of the most physical entities in all of creation—breaks down Jesus's body, and our digestive systems send bits and molecules of the God-human throughout our blood vessels, into cells at the far-most regions of our bodies. We are physically affected and spiritually nourished by this binary-busting reality. I know I'm using the word "literally" too much here, but our Catholic faith is literally birthed from the busted binary of spirit and flesh. The concept of Jesus as binary-buster begs so many questions. If the incarnation of Jesus resists the spirit/flesh binary, how does my body do the same? Our bodies inhabit a complex reality that cannot be reduced to binaries.

BINARY-BUSTING AS CHRISTIAN TRADITION

Jesus's mission to resist the binary may sound like a modern take on an ancient story, but I'm convinced that the seed of this reality has always been there in the texts of our faith. The seed has been germinating for millennia, and the implications are massive (and yes, the pun is always intended). Patrilie's words—the incarnation of Jesus resists the binary—were the water and sunlight I needed to help the seed grow, and now I can hardly believe I haven't noticed it before. And as the seed sprouted and poked its head above the soil, I reached back into my grad school course on literary theory and pulled out what I knew about binaries, power structures, structuralism, deconstruction, and various twentieth-century philosophers.

This is a major oversimplification, but structuralism sees binary opposition as fundamental to organizing our world (promoted by thinkers like Levi-Strauss and Lacan), while deconstructionism challenges binary oppositions by inverting and subverting them (promoted by thinkers like Michel Foucault and Jacques Derrida). A binary can express a power structure in this order: more powerful/less powerful. Or maybe "It is better to be A than B."

In other words, language matters—it shapes our very reality. For example, consider what lengths actors have their agents go to in order to ensure top billing for a movie poster or end credits. Language matters because it's how we communicate, deeper than even at the word level. With language, we categorize, applaud, accuse, acquit, and condemn. That being the case, let's play a little game. What does it feel like when we switch the order on our binaries? Take our default of male/female. If I flip the words and try to say "female/male" out loud, I subconsciously hesitate because of how odd it feels. I have been conditioned (like 99.9 percent of you) to the default that men come first, in language and in practice. Women are second. Nonbinary people aren't seen to exist in this either/or situation. Reversing the words enables me to confront things I may not have noticed before. Foolish/wise—when would it ever be better to be foolish than wise? Fat/thin—if you even hint at this, people lose their damn minds. Culturally, we aren't allowed to even consider doing this thought exercise in public because it is taboo to glorify "ob*sity" in any way, shape, or form. (Pun intended. Always. I use an asterisk to replace the letter e inside the word "ob*sity" because in the fat liberation community, we consider it a slur as it has been used as such in medical and nonmedical settings to denigrate and dehumanize fat bodies.)

Turning cultural expectations upside down is as old as God seeking relationship with humans. Even though humans have always lived by "might makes right," consider that God's affection was set on the Israelites not because they "were more numerous than other peoples, for [they] were the fewest of all peoples" (Deuteronomy 7:7, NIV). *It's better to be strong than weak.* This is a cultural touchstone for Westerners; we despise weakness. To flip the script and say, "It's better to be weak than strong" is incredibly countercultural. Even Western Christians believe strength is better than weakness, despite the Scriptures, which present weakness as better than strength (see the words of St. Paul in 2 Corinthians 12:10).

In fact, in the New Testament, there is an abundance of binary-flipping (especially in the writings of St. Paul). Consider the revolution that is Galatians 3:28: "There is no longer Jew or Greek, there is no longer slave or free, there is no longer male and female; for all of you are one in Christ Jesus" (NRSV).

And this one has so many—foolish/wise, weak/strong, chosen/rejected, nothingness/somethingness: "But God has chosen the foolish things of the world to put to shame the wise, and God has chosen the weak things of the world to put to shame the things which are mighty; and the base things of the world and the things that are despised, God has chosen, and the things which are not, to bring to nothing the things that are, that no flesh should glory in [God's] presence" (1 Corinthians 1:27-29, NIV). If we back up a few verses in that same chapter, we learn that not only is the incarnation a binary-buster, but so is the cross. "For the message of the cross is foolishness to those who are perishing, but to us who are being saved it is the power of God . . . Has not God made foolish the wisdom of this world?" (1:18-19).

The cross breaks the life/death binary and tells us that they are not opposed to each other but are partners in redemption. Even Jesus's people, the descendants of those chosen *because* of their weaknesses, were challenged by the thought that God's anointed one would not throw off foreign oppressors but would suffer actual death, a seeming defeat. If the Messiah is supposed to bring freedom by a military intervention against oppression, then the one called Jesus Christ is not only a fool but a failure. It would be akin to Moses dying before Pharaoh let God's people go. How could an oppressed people find true liberty through death?

The way that Paul puts it in Philippians, the desire of the one God is to bust the God/human, spirit/flesh, infinite/finite binary by God becoming a human . . . forever. In Philippians 2:1-4, Paul says that as children of God, we can love each other, seek unity of mind and spirit, and value one another above ourselves by rejecting the might-makes-right *modus operandi* of courting power (could we call this naked ambition?) and seeing success (could we call this the abundant life?) as a zero-sum game. A zero-sum game has winners and losers. It's a pie that can be cut into slices and consumed until there is nothing left. That's not the life that God creates for us. When I was a kid, my parents described it as a pie that, if you cut a piece and gave it away, you would turn around and find that there was still just as much pie left for everyone. Like when Jesus feeds the crowds with five loaves of bread and two little fish. And how Jesus shares his very self with us all over the world, every hour and every day, through the consecrated bread and wine.

RIPPLES IN THE POND

So when Patrilie articulated the truth of Jesus's binary-busting for me, it resonated. Have you ever taken a clear glass of water and run your finger around the edge faster and faster until you get music? The vibrations of the glass cause ripples in the water. Or have you skipped a stone in a pond and watched the water respond? There's a kerplunk, and the water is swept up into concentric circles traveling out from the center of its final destination. I felt like I had new language to describe what I had been learning for a long time: I don't have to live by the thin/fat, good/bad binary anymore, and when I throw myself into the pond (my body in its fullness with my larger-than-life personality—my whole self), the pond will resound and ripple because I exist. And that is an objective good. And also an objectively good way to communicate what this book is about (see the ripples on the cover).

Jesus busted binaries, and his followers did the same after him (Acts 17:6, NKJV). To quote *The Mandalorian*: "This is the way." It looks different, people, but Jesus leads us to do the same as he did: set people free from the boxes and binaries so they may live in freedom, without fear. By resisting the thin-good/fat-bad binary, we are doing the same thing. This is the way!

Dieting is built on a binary, thin/fat, that upholds a power arrangement. The widely accepted concept of "thinner is better" helps create and uphold a size-based hierarchy called sizeism. It is accompanied by healthism, the idea that health is the goal of life. This system is made up of all our beliefs about bodies, their purposes, and how they connect to our identities, particularly within communities. Within a given space, the thinnest, trimmest person of a given gender is more highly regarded than their fellow counterparts, colleagues, or congregants. Most of the time, this sizeist ranking system percolates though our sacred spaces.

If we want to cultivate lives and physical spaces where Jesus's tradition of binary-busting is honored and people are set free, we must identify the binaries that our way of life upholds and begin to disentangle ourselves from them. By doing this, we recognize that life is not defined by binaries and that our bodies are beautifully complex.

PACKING LIST

- Identify the binaries you rely on to define your world.
  - For example, thin/fat, healthy/unhealthy, abled/disabled, clean/unclean
- Ask questions of the binaries:
  - Why do I believe it is better to be thin than to be fat?

- Why do I demand health from my body and lament when it is unhealthy?
- Do I believe that an abled person is more worthy than a disabled person?
- Do I categorize food as clean and unclean, and if so, is that a fair thing to do?

■ Acknowledge the ways you have let binaries shape your world unjustly.
  - For example, admit if you treat thin and healthy people better than fat and/or unhealthy people.

--- TOUCHSTONE ---

MY BODY IS BEAUTIFUL AND COMPLEX.

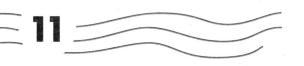

11

YOUR HEALTH IS NOT DETERMINED BY YOUR SIZE

Health: not equal to thinness, no matter what the prevailing culture says.

WHEN I WAS GROWING UP, visits to the doctor were dreaded because I knew it was inevitable that the doctor would want to talk to me about my weight. I never met a doctor who didn't equate my size to my health; they always assumed that I couldn't be healthy simply because I was in the 90 percent of the weight-to-height ratio for my age. Looking back now, I wasn't actually fat as a child, but I was bigger than all my peers, and my parents thought that meant I wasn't healthy. I visited doctor after doctor, my parents trying to find the secret to making me smaller. There was so much shame attached to being fat that we never used that word. "Big-boned" and "hefty" were the words of the day, before "plus size" became the norm. If you had told thirteen-year-old Amanda that people actually studied the reality of being fat in a world built for thinness, I would have laughed. Why would you study something so embarrassing? If people didn't want to be fat, I believed they should just follow all the diets and exercise regimens I was on, even though they didn't seem to be "working" for me. The news of an academic field called "fat studies" would have blown me away. Now I see that it's exactly what we need to combat the "size equals state of health" myth. Along with the work of dietitians like Evelyn Tribole and Elyse Resch (authors of *Intuitive Eating*), fat scholars have been empirically disproving that myth, along with many others, and normalizing the conversation around fatness in the academy and beyond.

FAT STUDIES

Fat studies emerged as an academic field at the beginning of the twenty-first century. (Fat British activist Charlotte Cooper thinks it should be called fat *American* studies, though, because it tends to push non-American realities to its margins.) In 2009, New York University Press published *The Fat Studies Reader*, edited by Esther Rothblum, a women's studies professor at San Diego State University, and Sondra Solovay, a law professor. Marilyn Wann wrote the foreword, and the collection of fat activists and authors is substantial. Shortly thereafter, in 2012, the *Fat Studies* academic journal debuted with Esther Rothblum as editor. It originally came out twice a year, but since 2017, there have been three issues annually.

Charlotte Cooper's own 2016 addition to fat studies, *Fat Activism: A Radical Social Movement*, resists the traditional approach to the field, if something as emergent as fat studies can have a "traditional approach." *Fat Activism* is a welcome addition, providing a treasure trove of firsthand accounts of the fat liberation movement on both sides of the pond. The aspect I enjoy most about Cooper's work is her insistence that the most important fat activism doesn't happen at NAAFA meetings or in academic research focused on ob*sity policy but in everyday acts of rebellion against fat phobia through countercultural choices in art, clothing, community, and self-expression.[2] The researchers and scholars in the field of fat studies are making a true difference in the way that fat people around the world are treated, but the task ahead is huge. My experience with COVID-19 is one example of where things need to improve.

SICK WHILE FAT
The Year from Hell

Scene: Under a bridge in Central Park

A large creature with two sets of horns, red skin, and cloven hooves approaches a woman who has an expectant look on her face.

"Satan?" she asks earnestly.

"Two-zero-two-zero?" he responds.

Breathlessly, she replies, "Call me Twenty-twenty."

Did you see this ad in the waning months of the worst year in recent history? A match made in hell, perfectly captured in a Match.com commercial. Satan and the year 2020 start dating, and the happy couple frolic through an empty New York City, shut down due to the coronavirus pandemic. They see movies in wide, empty theaters; work out in empty gyms; steal gobs and gobs of toilet paper, living our best lives instead of us. I suspect a past version of myself might not have found this ad very funny. But 2020 Amanda had seen some things. She was ready for this kind of humor. Much to my family's chagrin, I watched it repeatedly and shared it with all my friends.

"We are living in historic times" is a phrase we heard a lot in 2020, along with variations replacing "historic" with "unprecedented" and "extraordinary." Over and over and over again.

In future generations, I'm sure the year 2020 will stick in schoolchildren's memories of the world's timeline, much like I have 1066—the Battle of Hastings—stuck in mine. I can't even tell you what happened at the Battle of Hastings, but I know it took place in 1066. Real useful, y'all. But I'm sure that future kids will know this year as the year that the videoconferencing platform Zoom captured a beastly portion of market share and went on to dominate the world, forcing us all into a real-life Dilbert comic where our cubicles are our bedrooms and we can never leave even if we try. But I digress.

One Friday morning, my nose started running, and my body felt weaker than usual. A drive-by nasal swab that afternoon confirmed my suspicion: it was COVID-19, and I had unknowingly exposed my husband, my kids, and possibly my parents. Thus began the hardest two months of our lives. If you were to take the classic show *Wonder Years* and set it in a predominantly Jewish Philly suburb in the 1980s and add in ten times the dysfunction and crass humor, you'd get ABC's *The Goldbergs*. Written by Adam Goldberg, it's a hilarious fictionalized account of his growing pains as the nerdy, silver-screen-obsessed youngest child of three. Adam's father, Murray, portrayed by fat actor Jeff Garlin, is something else. The minute he walks in the door after working at his furniture store, he immediately sheds his slacks and, in his tighty whities, proceeds to his recliner in front of the family television.

After testing positive for COVID-19, I tried to emulate Murray Goldberg as much as I reasonably could, taking up permanent residence in my Sam's Club leather recliner and avoiding all restrictive clothing. All six of us—my husband, Zachary; our four young kids; and I—were infected after my positive test. But after a week, everyone else got better, while I sat pantsless and panting, in that recliner. It kept getting harder to breathe.

Eight days after my diagnosis and a course of both antibiotics and steroids, my oxygen saturation continued to decrease. If hospitals weren't inundated with sick people because of the pandemic, I probably would have gone to the ER sooner. When I finally went, my oxygen stats were at 72 (supposed to be about 97–99). They triaged me in an isolation room, all personnel covered in head-to-toe hazmat style, and began both supplemental oxygen and an IV. (I'm a hard stick, so that was fun. Not.) Time lost its meaning. COVID-19 had affected my perception of reality, so much so that I really believed I wasn't that sick. I expected them to prescribe me breathing treatments and send me back home to heal. When the ER doc told me I was going to stay the night, I had no idea that the next forty days would be the nightmare of my life.

A Different Kind of Pilgrimage

The nurse prepped me to be transferred, and when she asked me to put on my mask for transport, I was nonplussed. But when another staffer said that transport protocol on my stretcher required me to be covered head to toe in a white sheet, I panicked. It was 3:00 p.m. I had eaten nothing before coming to the ER five hours earlier. Mind you, this was after a week of not having energy even to eat much beyond saltines and juice. By the time I made it to my room, I was too weak to get from my bed to the bathroom. It was only about seven feet away, but neither my energy level nor my oxygen leash would allow it. I tried once, taking off my oxygen cannula so I could sit down, but I almost passed out from lack of oxygen. The bedside commode they brought me had arms for stability. Unfortunately, the arms did not give my large backside enough girth, so I was painfully suspended by the arms above the toilet seat while I defecated. Unsurprisingly, I made a mess, and with whatever awareness I had left, I was humiliated when the nurse came in and saw. It took them several hours, but they finally found a commode that could accommodate my body. And on top of all that, I was prohibited from using my continuous positive airway pressure (CPAP), a machine that keeps me breathing well while I sleep.

I was undone. My empty stomach and the ignored requests for food convinced me that they saw my fat body and thought I had the reserves to make it until dinner trays were served. Now I can see that this was the onset of paranoia, a symptom connected with COVID-19. At the time, though, it was real to me. I believed they were denying me food because I was fat. And it struck my heart with terror. Even when they did bring me trays of food, the portions were not enough for me. Biologically speaking, a fat body goes through more energy a day than a smaller body. I wasn't getting enough to sustain me.

Thankfully, that night they moved me to a room where it was safe to use my CPAP, and with me came my bariatric bedside toilet. My fat body was mostly accommodated, so I was resting a little easier in spirit, but my body was still fighting with all its might against COVID-19, and it didn't seem to have enough in it to defeat the disease.

The morning of October 27 (I remember the date because my daughter turned five that day), after being served breakfast on a lovely Styrofoam tray, I pulled out my Sharpies and started to write notes to each of my kids. I didn't know if I would ever see them again, and I wanted them to know how much Mama loved them. That was the day I got transferred to the ICU. I was too weak to speak, so I wrote a note in crudely drawn letters and sent a photo of it to my husband. They covered me in a white sheet again and transported me to intensive care. Making it to the ER and then to the ICU were significant milestones on my COVID-19 journey. For the next month, nobody knew if my pilgrimage would bring me back home, into the arms of my family, or to the loving arms of God in heaven.

My time in the ICU was fraught, and honestly, at the risk of sounding dramatic, I have no idea how much of what I remember is true. I was experiencing hallucinations where my medical conditioning shone through—I truly believed that I was experiencing what doctors had been trying to do to my body my whole life (make it smaller) and that people were trying to make my life not matter. I dreamed I was subjected to forced weight-loss surgery and lost half of myself. I believed that the nurses were intentionally not giving me enough nutrients through my feeding tube because they wanted to help me lose weight. It was traumatic, to say the least, and my nurses, despite their good intentions and amazing medical skills, just couldn't understand. I wasn't able to communicate the terrors I was experiencing, which made me feel isolated, alone, and scared.

I was so angry and confused, but something miraculous happened in my hallucinations. One day in the ICU, I had an unusual dream about my body lacking the ability to communicate. I was in a long-term care facility in New York, with severe physical limitations that prevented me from speaking or moving on my own. As hard as I tried to communicate with the nursing staff that was caring for me, and as much as they loved me, I had so much to say that I just couldn't. I was in pain, but no one could help me. A man with a long beard came in the door, walked over to my bed, and held my hand. As soon as I saw him, the name Sharbel popped into my head. He knew what I was thinking and could see the pain I was in.

"Breathe, Amanda," Sharbel said to me. "Let your pain be your prayer. Even if they never know you're praying for them." It was hard to breathe; COVID-19 inflicts a particularly devastating type of pneumonia on the lungs. But I started to breathe deeply anyway. In. Out. Feeling the pain but embracing it instead of fearing it. And as much as I wanted the pain to go away, I noticed something mingled within it. Comfort . . . and maybe even some joy? It felt strange and sweet, like it was a secret between me and God. Both of us swirled together in the pain and in the comfort, a moment of divine solidarity in the midst of uncertainty and suffering. Just recounting it now brings me to tears. I was not alone. I am not alone. My life matters.

A few days later, after I had come back to myself, the psychotic episodes began to fade in their intensity. But some images lingered, particularly the image of Sharbel. His was not a face I had seen and identified before; I just knew his name when he held my hand. And the only other place I had encountered that name was on my Bradbury pilgrimage five years before, in that little family restaurant outside of Chicago. Little Sharbel, whose family's food had refreshed me at the end of my pilgrimage and left a mark on my soul. My fingers and hands were very weak and had little muscle tone after so long not being used, so it took some time before I could find a picture of Sharbel on the internet. But when I did, there he was—older but full-bearded and familiar. Months after leaving the hospital, when I learned that the name Sharbel means "the breath of Bel is good," I did a double take. In the languages of the ancient Near East, "Bel" was a title for God like "Lord" is today. So a saint whose name means "the breath of the Lord is good" came to me in a vision while I was hospitalized with a lung disease and taught me to pray by breathing in and out and offering my suffering as a prayer. It's an experience I will treasure forever on this pilgrimage, and as often as I think of it, I say a prayer for little Sharbel, who probably isn't so little anymore.

Fat people should be able to have faith in our medical system that it is not actively looking to harm them by making them smaller at any cost. I really believe that if medical fat phobia wasn't as deeply entrenched as I have experienced it to be, I would have suffered less in my darkest hours with COVID-19. Uprooting medical fat phobia is a huge and multifaceted task, but it can begin in the doctor's office for an annual wellness visit. Below is a handout I created for the listeners of the *Fat & Faithful* podcast I cohosted with J. Nicole Morgan from 2017 through 2020. It provides a script for you to take with you into your doctor's office visits, which you can copy and hand to your primary care provider or read to them.

Important information regarding my treatment for use by my primary care provider, specialists, and their staffs

My medical history involves several instances of being treated in an unprofessional manner by health-care providers. This causes anxiety related to health-care appointments, so I ask that for this appointment, you observe the following guidelines:

- o I decline to be weighed at this appointment. If my care requires weight for correct dosage, I will consent to being weighed, but I do not wish to know the number. Please make a note on my chart, but I do not want to know the number under any circumstances.
- o I do not consent to discussions of treatment that involve weight loss. Research indicates that dieting fails 95 percent of patients and has harmful results for mental and physical health. I will not discuss treatment options that have a goal of weight loss or dieting.
- o I request treatment recommendations that are based on peer-reviewed research and are prescribed for patients in the normal range on the body mass index (BMI) chart. The medical issue I am here for has treatments that can be administered within the framework of health at every size. I want a treatment plan that deals with

---

the measurable indicators of my health that do not include weight.

If you are willing to consult with me according to these parameters, I am willing to continue this appointment so we can decide the best path forward for me and my health. If not, let us end this appointment respectfully so that I can pursue my health care with another provider.

Health at Every Size and Intuitive Eating

As many people come to realize the harm of diet culture, they want to leave dieting behind forever. This, however, is very hard when most of what we have been taught about bodies and health is connected to food rules and restrictions and making sure we are moving "enough." When we finally decide to leave diet culture, it can be scary because dieting has defined so much of our lives and given us a sense of control. It can feel intimidating to confront how our lifelong practices have perpetuated the lack of peace with food and our body.

Thankfully, two revolutionary frameworks can help us along this journey, HAES™ and Intuitive Eating (IE). These two frameworks lean into the reality that our bodies are trustworthy—if our bodies are in pain, we treat them with care, and if our bodies are hungry, we feed them. HAES is a way of looking at health holistically and through respect, critical awareness, and compassionate self-care, a framework popularized by Lindo Bacon, PhD, and Lucy Aphramor, PhD, RD.[3] The HAES framework recognizes that a person's weight and size are not reliable indicators of health and also that health is more than the absence of disease or pain in the body; health is multifaceted—including physical health, mental health, and emotional wellness—and is dependent on a just health-care system and an inclusive society. With a HAES mindset, you can see your health as more than simply your weight and the size of your body. It enables everyone— no matter the size or shape of their body—to pursue health as they need and desire, without aiming to lose weight or make themselves smaller.

The second revolutionary framework for finding peace with your body is Intuitive Eating, a set of principles developed by registered dietitians and eating disorder specialists Evelyn Tribole and Elyse Resch. Their book, *Intuitive Eating: A Revolutionary Anti-Diet*, is now available in its fourth edition, which states boldly on the cover that it is possible to "make peace with food, free yourself from chronic dieting forever, and rediscover the pleasures of eating." In its pages, Resch and Tribole take the reader through ten principles to reset how we have been taught to think about food and exercise. They explain how a diet mentality sabotages our entire relationship with our body, food, and exercise.

PACKING LIST

- Script for a weight-neutral doctor visit:

Important information regarding my treatment for use by my primary care provider, specialists, and their staffs

My medical history involves several instances of being treated in an unprofessional manner by health-care providers. This causes anxiety related to health-care appointments, so I ask that for this appointment, you observe the following guidelines:

- o I decline to be weighed at this appointment. If my care requires weight for correct dosage, I will consent to being weighed, but I do not wish to know the number. Please make a note on my chart, but I do not want to know the number under any circumstances.
- o I do not consent to discussions of treatment that involve weight loss. Research indicates that dieting fails 95 percent of patients and has harmful results for mental and physical health. I will not discuss treatment options that have a goal of weight loss or dieting.
- o I request treatment recommendations that are based on peer-reviewed research and are prescribed for patients in the normal range on the BMI chart. The medical issue I am here for has treatments that can be administered within the framework of health at every size. I want a treatment plan that deals with the measurable indicators of my health that do not include weight.

If you are willing to consult with me according to these parameters, I am willing to continue this appointment so we can decide the best path forward for me and my health. If not, let us end this appointment respectfully so that I can pursue my health care with another provider.

■ Health at Every Size™ and Intuitive Eating
Ask your health-care provider if they are familiar
with the Health at Every Size™ and/or Intuitive
Eating frameworks for their patients in larger
bodies. Use this script as an example:

Doctor, are you familiar with the Health at Every
Size™ or the Intuitive Eating approaches to health
and wellness? Health at Every Size™ focuses on more
reliable indicators of health than weight, like blood
pressure or blood sugar levels. I would like to know
action steps I can take that are not focused on losing
weight but that help me regulate these numbers in
my life. Intuitive Eating helps me work with my body's
cues and to engage in joyful movement so that we are
in harmony rather than in a constant psychological
battle from forced dieting and exercise.

To learn more about these paradigms,
you can visit these sites for more information:
haescommunity.org and https://www.intuitiveeating
.org/what-is-intuitive-eating-tribole/.

TOUCHSTONE

> # MY HEALTH IS NOT DETERMINED BY MY SIZE.

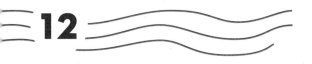

12

THE WORLD NEEDS MORE OF YOU

More: a greater or additional amount or degree of something.

IN 2009, *TIME MAGAZINE* WRITER DAN FLETCHER wrote an article about NAAFA's fortieth anniversary, giving some history about the fat-in, Bill Fabrey, and the Fat Underground. The article is about the same length as the one that appeared in the *New York Times* in the summer of 1967, which existed in mere obscurity, buried in section L, crowded by ads for Broadway shows. And while it's true that I accessed both from my computer in East Texas, one is preserved for history as an image in the *New York Times* archives; the other (Fletcher's) exists like any modern online article—littered with links, making it challenging to navigate without clicking on the click bait and paid content. But the angering part about that difference is all of the hyperlinks to other "related" *TIME* articles: "First Comes Love, Then Comes Obesity?" and "Why Are Southerners So Fat?" and "Brazilian Obesity: The Big Girl from Ipanema." Hey, *TIME Magazine*, your anti-fat bias is showing.

While there is plenty of fat stigma, body shaming, and concern trolling still happening, fat representation is more visible than ever, in media and in print. The adaptation of Lindy West's memoir *Shrill* starred fat comedian Aidy Bryant, of *Saturday Night Live* fame—one of the first shows with a fat protagonist not centered on a weight-loss journey. Lizzo has blown our minds with her phenomenal musical talent paired with her in-your-face radical acceptance of her body. Priscila Arias, also known as La-Fatshionista on Instagram, reaches her more than five hundred thousand IG followers with fashion and body liberation messages. Fat liberation has come so far from where we started.

And we still have so far to go. Although the movement has always wanted to be an inclusive place of intersectionality, there are many more stories and so much more wisdom than the majority-white, female voices that have been published since the movement's start in the 1960s. The foundational beliefs of fat liberation—the dignity of every body no matter its size, the right to self-determination, and the right to accessibility—overlap and intersect with the vision of disability activists, queer activists, Black activists and other activists of color, and more. If you're not following authors and activists like Sonya Renee Taylor (*The Body Is Not an Apology*) and Virgie Tovar (*You Have the Right to Remain Fat*), change that ASAP. The history of fat liberation is still to be written, and it is an intersectional one. People of every identity are learning to lean into their truest selves, whether they be queer, disabled, fat, BIPOC, or any combination of the above. We are all learning together, and it is an honor to travel with you, no matter who you are or how you identify.

As our journey together draws to a close, I want to leave you with a bag full of skipping stones to make ripples in every pond you pass out in the field. Look back at the touchstones we have picked up and put in our pocket along the way. All bodies are good bodies. Your today body is good. Fat is not a bad word. It's okay to be fat. You have the right to take up space. You can stop shrinking yourself. Your body is a storyteller. Curiosity is your body's friend. Your body is your home. Your body is beautiful and complex. Your health is not determined by your size. And, finally, the world needs more of you. And by "world," I mean everybody you come in contact with, and the people who they come in contact with, and the people who they come in contact with. And so on. Your life, lived to the full, matters—and not just for you.

One day I checked my Instagram and saw I had been tagged in a photo by someone I didn't know. The story I read in its caption brought tears to my eyes, and with permission I am sharing it with you. The image was of several potted succulents of various colors, shapes, and sizes in three rows, with the words "WRONG WAY TO HAVE A BODY" written in small block letters in between the lines.

The poster, a school counselor in training named Mary, wrote the following:

A couple days ago as I finished working with a group of 3rd graders, one of the girls hung back while I cleaned off the table.

"Ms. Mary, can I talk to you?"

"Always! What's up?" I said.

"One of the boys called me fat, and it really hurt my feelings."

My heart sank. Everything in me wanted to say, "I'm so sorry he said that. You are not fat. Don't listen to him." But instead, I asked myself what I needed someone to say to me when I was in 3rd grade (or 1st grade, really) when other kids called me fat. I told her, "I'm so sorry he said that. That must have really hurt. Can I tell you the truth, though? The truth is, your body is a good body. Your body is exactly as it's supposed to be. You're growing and changing, and it's really awesome that your body is able to do that, don't you think? Other people may have opinions about your body or someone else's body, but the most important thing you can remember is that all bodies are good bodies."

She smiled. I told her again, "Your body is good. Your body is exactly how it's supposed to be. Nothing anyone else may say will ever change that. Your body is good." [. . .] I know . . . I was that 8-year-old. The first time I remember being called fat, I was 5 years old. I began throwing food away from my lunch at 5 years old, because of what other kids said to me. And the bullying never stopped. I needed someone to tell me what I told this sweet kiddo today. ALL bodies are GOOD bodies.

Mary's story hit me hard in the feels, because this is my dream: for the little fat girls in elementary school to be given this message every damn day, and for every day after that.

It's not just for the little girls in elementary school bathrooms crying their eyes out because they were picked last again for teams. "The world needs more of you" is a message for every beautiful human in this gigantic, beautiful world. So, yes, reader—I'm looking straight at you. You. I need more of you. You need more of you. The world needs more of you. Now get out there, skip some stones, and be your full self—and let the ripples change the world today. I'll leave you with the words of a foremother of fat liberation, Judy Freespirit: "The story of fat women's liberation is just beginning."

PACKING LIST

- Fill the world with more of you, and then some more.
  - Stop trying to make yourself smaller, body and soul.
  - It's not letting yourself go; it's letting yourself be.
  - Let yourself take up space.
  - Wear what you want.
  - Eat what you want.
  - Stand up for yourself and for others who are marginalized.
  - Your freedom will ripple out around you, changing more lives than you can ever imagine.

TOUCHSTONE

THE WORLD NEEDS MORE OF ME.

ACKNOWLEDGMENTS

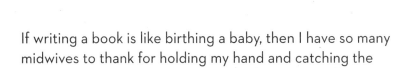

If writing a book is like birthing a baby, then I have so many midwives to thank for holding my hand and catching the creation I've pushed out. (Too visual? Sorry, not sorry.)

To my agent, Keely Boeving, and my editor, Lisa Kloskin—without you, this book would have stayed in my head. Thank you for encouraging me to draw it out. To my writing coaches, Ruth Buchanan and Jessica Kantrowitz, y'all really have a gift for helping writers find their words and their direction. To the design team at Broadleaf—this book cover helped shape my writing, especially the ripples in the pond; you made this a better book by your work.

To my friends who have listened to me, encouraged me, and celebrated me whenever I was in great despair or great joy because of this manuscript—thank you. To the members of All Bodies Are Good bodies, especially my admin team—Stephanie Ilderton, Micah Emerson, Sandy Shackelford, Fayelle Ewuakye, Valerie Bojarski, and J. Nicole Morgan. Nicole, specifically, thank you for *Fat & Faithful*. Your incarnated advocacy and leadership made a way for this book to exist. I am the woman and the writer I am today because of you, your writing, and your friendship.

To my Twitter pastor, Rev. Heidi Carrington Heath (@revfemme), and my Instagram pastor, Rev. Lizzie—y'all need to know how much your prayers and blessings formed my heart along the journey of writing this book.

To my best friend, Kelley, thank you for your support and cheerleading.

To my husband, Zachary, for his stalwart belief in and support of my mission that everyone can know that their bodies are good. To my family, especially my kids, who keep me honest on bad body-image days—"All bodies are good bodies, Mom!"

Most of all, thank you to the God who is not afraid of me taking up space, the one who says to each of us, "You are enough. You are not too much. The world needs more of you."

APPENDIX A: FAT LEXICON

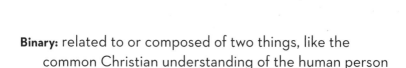

Binary: related to or composed of two things, like the common Christian understanding of the human person as body and soul or flesh and spirit.

Body Positivity: originally used by fat liberationists as shorthand for their work. Today it has been co-opted by non-fat people and corporations as a focus on feeling good about your body rather than focusing on freeing people from anti-fat oppression.

Body Shame: the invisible burden of embarrassment, grief, and disappointment caused by a misplaced concern that your body doesn't measure up to someone's ideal body standards.

Diet Culture: a cultural influence built on a fundamentally flawed way of looking at bodies, which upholds a body hierarchy based on thinness as good and fatness as bad. It is inextricably linked with other social hierarchies like race and class, and it encourages marginalization of BIPOC, the fat community, those with disabilities, those with chronic illnesses, non-male genders, those in poverty, and more.

Fat: not a bad word; a morally neutral way to describe a body; an accessibility issue.

Fat Hospitality: the act of creating welcome private and public spaces for fat bodies, including adequate seating, access to facilities, and an atmosphere of fat acceptance.

Fat Liberation: a freedom movement, birthed in the 1960s, emphasizing natural body diversity and embracing fatness and the right of fat people to dignified treatment in every area of life. Fat liberation tears down systemic fat oppression at every level: personal, interpersonal, community-based, and structural. It addresses the need for and the obstacles against the inclusion of fat people and creates a world where it truly is okay to be fat.

Gluttony: consumption that harms your neighbor (J. Nicole Morgan).

Good: to be desired or approved of; the quality of something that fulfills its purpose.

Health: not equal to thinness, no matter what the prevailing culture says.

Intuition: a creature's natural ability to sense its dietary, sleep, movement, and emotional needs and to reasonably achieve them; how our body talks to us.

More: a greater or additional amount or degree of something, particularly of yourself.

Politics: what happens when bodies take up space near each other, the fallout of this, and its organization.

APPENDIX B: COMPLETE KNAPSACK PACKING LIST

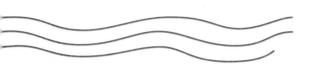

CHAPTER 1
- Knapsack
- Sturdy hiking shoes
- Clothing with pockets
- Open heart and mind

CHAPTER 2
- My fat imagination. I actively employ my imagination so that I can envision who I want to be, where I want to go, or how I want to be treated. I can let my imagination run as wild as I want because I am the one making decisions for me. I've included the *who, what, where, how,* and *why* that exist in my fat imagination. It doesn't have to be in list form like mine is—you could make a vision board, make a painting, construct a PowerPoint presentation, or do a timeline in memes.
  - *What I want to experience:* a world where every person is treated with dignity and compassion no matter their size, shape, ability, or level of health.

- *Who I want to be:* like the woman that C. S. Lewis describes in *The Great Divorce,* life and joy overflowing and spreading out around my fat body, spilling onto others.
- *Where I want to go:* to a place where I am completely free to exist in my today body, where body size does not determine my worth or my level of access to public and private spaces.
- *How I want to get there:* with a radical belief in the goodness of my body even with its weaknesses . . . even perhaps because of its weaknesses.
- *Why I want to go there:* to bring others along with me as we pursue peace and freedom so that we can change the world with our fat imaginations.

CHAPTER 3

- Challenging fat stereotypes:
  - In media portrayals, ask:
    - o Did you notice any fat people in the movie?
    - o How are they portrayed: good or bad, nice or evil, simple or complex?
    - o Do you know any fat people in real life?
    - o Are they like the fat characters in the movie?
    - o Are they different than the fat characters in the movie?
  - In negative language, ask:
    - o How can I communicate my feelings and needs without denigrating fatness?
    - o Do I make fatness the butt of jokes, even self-deprecating ones?

- In terms of accessibility, ask:
  - o Are the places I frequent (work, restaurants, stores, places of worship, etc.) friendly to fat bodies?
  - o How can I use my voice to advocate for fat bodies?
    - Ask for inclusive seating with armless and sturdy seats.
    - Ask for sizes larger than my own to be stocked.

CHAPTER 4

- Liberating the oppressed: how to do this for yourself and others to create a world where it is okay to be fat. Examine the narratives and history around you. Ask yourself:
  - What about this narrative needs to be different in order to be truly just? What gems of wisdom are here?
  - How does this change my life?
  - How does this bring freedom to oppressed people?
  - With whom do I need to share this?

CHAPTER 5

- The Fat Girl's Bill of Rights: Try standing in front of a mirror and speaking these rights to yourself in the first person. You may experience some internal resistance at first but repeat them over and over again until they feel true and deeply rooted in your soul.
  1. I have the right to exist in my body today.
  2. I have the right to take up space.

3. I have the right to eat the foods I want to eat.
4. I have the right to wear whatever I want.
5. I have the right to compassionate and informed fat-aware medical care.
6. I have the right to maintain boundaries over my body.
7. I have the right to move my body in any way I choose.
8. I have the right to live a public life without ridicule or abuse because of my body.
9. I have the right to reject diet culture.
10. I have the right to embrace the mystery of my body.

CHAPTER 6

- Questions to identify diet culture:
  - Does it convey the goodness of every body, or does it value thin and trim bodies over fat ones?
  - Does this hold all genders to the same standard?
  - Is this accessible to people despite their financial circumstances?
  - Does this make room for disabled and chronically ill bodies or uphold a skewed and ableist vision of health?
  - Does this recognize the roles that genetics, ability, class, and gender play in body size, or does it promise to control body size?
  - Who stands to benefit from this financially, socially, or morally?
  - Does this inspire body acceptance and freedom or body shame?

CHAPTER 7

- ■ My body is a storyteller: I need the right questions about the story my body is telling.
    - What story is my body telling?
    - How does that story differ from the one I believe about my body?
    - How can I listen more to my body's good story, even if pain comes along with that story?
    - Does the idea of pilgrimage help you see your body's story more clearly?
- ■ Sit or stand in front of a mirror. Look at yourself with tender eyes. What story do you see? Is that a true story? If not, what is the true story? What lies have you been believing about the story your body is telling?

CHAPTER 8

- ■ How to climb out of the body-shame spiral. Learn to identify the landmarks of the spiral:
    1. Triggering Event
    2. Response
    3. Observation
    4. Wishful Thinking
    5. Assigning Blame
    6. Negative Projection
    7. The Pit of Despair
        - Insert curiosity at whatever level you find yourself at. Ask good questions of your responses and emotions. Over time, you will learn to recognize the shame spiral close to its start, and often you can more easily prevent

yourself from slipping down the path, climbing out from wherever you find yourself in it.

- Questions and statements to use when the conversation turns to fatness, whether that happens at home or in public:
  - Make no assumptions.
    - The first time my daughter called me fat, she had no idea that the term could be offensive. When children ask loud questions or make comments about bodies, make sure you understand their mindset before offering a corrective. Kids aren't fat phobic until they are taught to be.
  - Approach with curiosity.
    - I try to respond with a question that needs more than a yes/no answer, like "Oh, yeah? What does that mean to you?" I let the child explain what the word "fat" means to them, and then I go from there with a question such as "Do you think it's okay to be fat? Why or why not?"
  - Examine personal biases.
    - The children around me will pick up on the way I view my body and other bodies. I must continue to work on my own bias against fatness so that it does not transfer to them.
  - Reinforce truth.

    The barrage of diet culture negativity will threaten to overwhelm any fat-positive foundation I am laying with the kids in my life, so I almost always end conversations about bodies with this call and response:

Me: And what do we say about bodies? (wait)
Me and child: All bodies are good bodies!
  o Your own call and response could be any
    variation of this truth. Come up with it in your
    community, whether that's in your family, in your
    classroom, or in children's church.

CHAPTER 9

- Use your imagination to enter the door of your body
  and look around. What parts of you do you need to
  embrace? What rooms surprise you? What rooms do
  you want to feel more at home in?
- Once you're at home in your body, check out the
  neighborhood! Finding fat community is vital,
  particularly when it comes to specialized communities
  on social media such as:
  - Fat fashion
  - Fat sex
  - Fat romance
  - Fat accessibility
  - Fat-aware medical care
  - General fat community
  - My Facebook group, All Bodies Are Good Bodies,
    is a good place to start!

CHAPTER 10

- Identify the binaries you rely on to define your world.
  - For example, thin/fat, healthy/unhealthy, abled/
    disabled, clean/unclean.
- Ask questions of the binaries:
  - Why do I believe it is better to be thin than to be fat?

- Why do I demand health from my body and lament when it is unhealthy?
- Do I believe that an abled person is more worthy than a disabled person?
- Do I categorize food as clean and unclean, and if so, is that a fair thing to do?
■ Acknowledge the ways you have let binaries shape your world unjustly.
- For example, admit if you treat thin and healthy people better than fat and/or unhealthy people.

CHAPTER 11
■ Script for a weight-neutral doctor visit:

Important information regarding my treatment for use by my primary care provider, specialists, and their staffs

My medical history involves several instances of being treated in an unprofessional manner by health-care providers. This causes anxiety related to health-care appointments, so I ask that for this appointment, you observe the following guidelines:

o I decline to be weighed at this appointment. If my care requires weight for correct dosage, I will consent to being weighed, but I do not wish to know the number. Please make a note on my chart, but I do not want to know the number under any circumstances.
o I do not consent to discussions of treatments that involve weight loss. Research indicates

---

that dieting fails 95 percent of patients and has harmful results for mental and physical health. I will not discuss treatment options that have a goal of weight loss or dieting.

o I request treatment recommendations that are based on peer-reviewed research and are prescribed for patients in the normal range on the BMI chart. The medical issue I am here for has treatments that can be administered within the framework of health at every size. I want a treatment plan that deals with the measurable indicators of my health that do not include weight.

If you are willing to consult with me according to these parameters, I am willing to continue this appointment so we can decide the best path forward for me and my health. If not, let us end this appointment respectfully so that I can pursue my healthcare with another provider.

- Health at Every Size™ and Intuitive Eating
  Ask your health-care provider if they are familiar with the Health at Every Size™ and/or Intuitive Eating frameworks for their patients in larger bodies. Use this script as an example:
  Doctor, are you familiar with the Health at Every Size™ or the Intuitive Eating approaches to health and wellness? Health at Every Size™ focuses on more reliable indicators of health than weight,

like blood pressure or blood sugar levels. I would like to know action steps I can take that are not focused on losing weight but that help me regulate these numbers in my life. Intuitive Eating helps me work with my body's cues and to engage in joyful movement so that we are in harmony rather than in a constant psychological battle from forced dieting and exercise.

To learn more about these paradigms, you can visit these sites for more information: haescommunity.org and https://www.intuitiveeating .org/what-is-intuitive-eating-tribole/.

CHAPTER 12

- Fill the world with more of you, and then some more.
  - Stop trying to make yourself smaller, body and soul.
  - It's not letting yourself go; it's letting yourself be.
  - Let yourself take up space.
  - Wear what you want.
  - Eat what you want.
  - Stand up for yourself and for others who are marginalized.
  - Your freedom will ripple out around you, changing more lives than you can ever imagine.

APPENDIX C: TOUCHSTONES

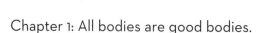

Chapter 1: All bodies are good bodies.
Chapter 2: My today body is good.
Chapter 3: "Fat" is not a bad word.
Chapter 4: It's okay to be fat.
Chapter 5: I have the right to take up space.
Chapter 6: I can stop shrinking myself.
Chapter 7: My body is a trustworthy storyteller.
Chapter 8: Curiosity is my body's friend.
Chapter 9: My body is my home.
Chapter 10: My body is beautiful and complex.
Chapter 11: My health is not determined by my size.
Chapter 12: The world needs more of me.

NOTES

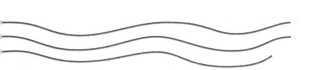

CHAPTER 1

1. This overlapping and compounding is known as *intersectionality*, a term defined by Black feminist scholar Kimberlé Crenshaw in 1989, explaining how a person's identity is more complex when that person is a part of more than one marginalized group. Crenshaw contends that a Black woman's experience is not merely the sum of her experience as a woman added to her experience of being Black but that those two marginalized identities overlap, creating a more complex reality.

CHAPTER 3

1. Valerie Bojarski (@theabundanttherapist), "FAT is not a bad word," Instagram caption, June 16, 2021, https://www.instagram.com/p /CQMBgPcrlhl/?utm_source=ig_web_copy_link.
2. Marilynn Wann, foreword to *The Fat Studies Reader*, by Esther D. Rothblum and Sondra Solovay (New York: New York University Press, 2009), xii.

CHAPTER 4

1. Tim Gunn, "Designers Refuse to Make Clothes to Fit American Women. It's a Disgrace," *Washington Post*, September 8, 2016, https://www.washingtonpost.com/posteverything/wp/2016/09/08 /tim-gunn-designers-refuse-to-make-clothes-to-fit-american-women -its-a-disgrace/.

2. Louis G. Iasilli, "The Pre-Marital Blood Test Law," *St. John's Law Review* 13, no. 1 (November 1938), https://scholarship.law.stjohns.edu /cgi/viewcontent.cgi?article=5629&context=lawreview.

CHAPTER 5

1. Lisa Schoenfielder and Barb Wiser, eds., *Shadow on a Tightrope: Writings by Women on Fat Oppression* (San Francisco: Aunt Lute Books, 1983), 55, from essay "Fat Woman and Women's Fear of Fat" by the Fat Underground, written by Lynn Mabel-Lois and Aldebaran.
2. Charlotte Cooper, *Fat Activism: A Radical Social Movement* (Bristol: HammerOn Press, 2016), 115.
3. Cooper, *Fat Activism*, 114.
4. Preface, Shadow on a Tightrope.
5. Judy Freespirit and Aldebaran, "Fat Liberation Manifesto," in *Shadow on a Tight Rope: Writings by Women on Fat Oppression*, eds. Lisa Schoenfielder and Barb Wieser (Iowa: Aunt Lute Book, 1983), 52–53.
6. Sara Golda Bracha Fishman, "Life in the Fat Underground," *Radiance Online: The Magazine for Large Women* (Winter 1998), http://www. radiancemagazine.com/issues/1998/winter_98/fat_underground.html.
7. Fishman, "Life in the Fat Underground."
8. Fishman, "Life in the Fat Underground."
9. Judy Freespirit and Aldebaran, "Fat Liberation Manifesto," *Off Our Backs* 9, no. 4 (1979): 18, www.jstor.org/stable/25773035.

CHAPTER 6

1. Amy Erdman Farrell, *Fat Shame: Stigma and the Fat Body in American Culture* (New York: New York University Press, 2011), 4. Emphasis mine.
2. Long Ge et al., "Comparison of Dietary Macronutrient Patterns of 14 Popular Named Dietary Programmes for Weight and Cardiovascular Risk Factor Reduction in Adults: Systematic Review and Network Meta-analysis of Randomized Trials," *BMJ* 369 (2020): m696; Kevin D. Hall and Scott Kahan, "Maintenance of Lost Weight and Long-Term Management of Obesity," *Medical Clinics of North America* 102, no. 1 (2018): 183–197.
3. Vanessa A. Diaz, Arch G. Mainous 3rd, and Charles J. Everett, "The Association between Weight Cycling and Mortality: Results from a

Population-based Cohort Study," *Journal of Community Health* 30, no. 3 (2005): 153–165.

4. "Report: Economic Costs of Eating Disorders," https://www.hsph.harvard.edu/striped/report-economic-costs-of-eating-disorders/.
5. G. C. Patton et al., "Onset of Adolescent Eating Disorders: Population-based Cohort Study Over 3 Years," *BMJ* 318, no. 7186 (1999): 765–768.
6. "Homepage," http://morelove.helpdocsonline.com/home.

CHAPTER 7

1. Richard Rohr's *Another Name for Every Thing* podcast, episode 1 "Christ-Soaked World," February 24, 2019.

CHAPTER 8

1. "Bread," symbolism of, Encyclopedia.com.

CHAPTER 9

1. Quoted in Charlotte Cooper, *Fat Activism: A Radical Social Movement* (Bristol: HammerOn Press), 141.
2. Charlotte Cooper, "Revisiting BBC Open Space: Fat Women Are Here to Stay," On her ObesityTimebomb blog, May 11, 2011, https://obesitytimebomb.blogspot.com/2011/05/revisiting-bbc-open-space-fat-women.html.
3. Cooper, *Fat Activism*, 146.
4. "Why Wendy's Is Facing Campus Protests (It's About the Tomatoes," *New York Times*, July 3, 2019, https://www.nytimes.com/2019/03/07/business/economy/wendys-farm-workers-tomatoes.html.

CHAPTER 11

1. Charlotte Cooper, "Maybe It Should Be Called Fat American Studies," in *The Fat Studies Reader*, eds. Esther Rothblum and Sondra Solovay (New York: New York University Press, 2009), 327–333.
2. Cooper, *Fat Activism*, 8.
3. HAEScommunity.com.